Praise for *Pain-Free Joints*

"*Pain-Free Joints* offers hope for more than just p
Sufferers may see improvement, or even a rever

"*Pain-Free Joints: 46 Simple Qigong Move* .*lealth*
and Prevention by Dr. Yang, Jwing-Ming .tion and
exercises to help treat arthritis. The book ackn ,es that both
Western medicine and Eastern medicine can be helpful, and suggests practical, clear, symptom-relieving steps for anyone suffering
from arthritis pain.

"The book is brief, well organized, and very clear, featuring exercises
that almost anyone can do. Yang discusses massage, acupuncture,
and cavity presses, and explains how each can be used to improve
the flow of qi, the natural energy that circulates throughout the
universe and also through the body. The book includes an infor-
mative and interesting comparison of Western and Eastern healing philosophy, focusing on treatment versus prevention. It does
not assume that one is right while the other is wrong, but instead
suggests that both can be used together to achieve overall good
health.

"Though the concepts being explained are quite complex, the book
is very easy to understand. Qigong, or the study of qi, is central to the
lessons, as is learning to affect how qi moves through the body. The
author explains that 'traditional Chinese physicians believe that
since the body's cells are alive, as long as there is a proper supply of qi, the physical damage can be repaired or even completely
rebuilt.' The book emphasizes the importance of understanding
the theory behind the suggested exercises and the need to make them
part of a lifelong practice. There is just enough basic information

to get started exploring this path to healing. There are also references for further study, and the book concludes with a very helpful glossary of Chinese terms.

"Abundant photographs demonstrate the recommended exercises, depicting a model performing each one. Despite being still, black-and-white forms, these images do a remarkable job of illustrating how to move through each activity. The accompanying descriptions are clear and easy to follow, with instructions on how to move the body through the exercise, how to breathe with the movement, and recommendations for the number of repetitions needed to be effective.

"Those who suffer from arthritis know that it can feel like an endless cycle of pain with little hope for improvement. What is perhaps most remarkable about *Pain-Free Joints* is that it offers hope for more than just pain management. Though the author warns that these exercises will take diligence and patience, with continued practice sufferers may see improvement, or even a reversal of their condition."

—Catherine Thureson, *Foreword Reviews*

"Dr. Yang's various qigong methods and techniques for arthritis are as thorough, and presumably effective, as his dedicated readers have grown to expect. What I especially appreciate is Dr. Yang's emphasis, and re-emphasis throughout this book, on the importance, not only of the *whats* and *hows* of his methods, but equally on the *whys*, which serve to empower his readers in a special way. In addition to providing meaning and understanding to the qigong healing techniques covered, the *whys* behind these methods serve to excite and motivate the practitioner's cortical brain, which plays a critically significant role in the mobilization of qi for self-healing purposes. This makes for a de facto blending of ancient qigong healing methods and modern neuroplasticity."

—John Loupos, MS, HSE, author of *The Sustainable You: Somatics and the Myth of Aging* and *Tai Chi Connections: Advancing Your Tai Chi Experience*; owner of the Pain and Mobility Clinic, Cohasset, Massachusetts

"As a classical Pilates instructor who works with students with arthritis every day, I was very interested in learning Dr. Yang's theories and techniques. That the book begins with explaining what arthritis is, the varying treatments of Chinese versus Western medicine, and how qigong specifically is effective in the maintenance of arthritis gives the reader the knowledge necessary for taking their wellness into their own hands. I can see this book being an invaluable tool that the reader will want to keep on hand to reference throughout their qigong practice."

—Sally Whitaker, Peak Pilates comprehensive instructor; studio manager at Studio on Main Pilates & Yoga, Independence, Missouri; owner of Move Forward Pilates

PAIN-FREE JOINTS

DR. YANG, JWING-MING

PAIN-FREE JOINTS

46 Simple Qigong Movements for Arthritis Healing and Prevention

YMAA Publication Center, Inc.
Wolfeboro, NH USA

YMAA Publication Center, Inc.
PO Box 480
Wolfeboro, New Hampshire, 03894
1-800-669-8892 • info@ymaa.com • www.ymaa.com

ISBN: 9781594395352 (print) • ISBN: 9781594395369 (ebook)

Edited by Leslie Takao and Doran Hunter
Cover design by Axie Breen
This book typeset in 11.5 pt. Minion Pro Regular
Typesetting by Westchester Publishing Services
Illustrations provided by the author unless otherwise noted.

POD0118

Publisher's Cataloging in Publication

Names: Yang, Jwing-Ming, 1946– author.
Title: Pain-free joints : 46 simple qigong movements for arthritis healing and
    prevention / Dr. Yang, Jwing-Ming.
Other titles: Yang, Jwing-Ming, 1946–. Arthritis relief.
Description: Wolfeboro, NH, USA : YMAA Publication Center, Inc., [2017] |
    "Abridgement of the larger book by Dr. Yang, Jwing-Ming titled 'Arthritis relief:
    Chinese qigong for healing and prevention.'" | Includes bibliographical references
    and index.
Identifiers: ISBN: 9781594395352 | 9781594395369 (ebook) | LCCN: 2017954710
Subjects: LCSH: Arthritis—Alternative treatment. | Arthritis—Exercise therapy. |
    Joints—Diseases—Alternative therapy. | Joints—Diseases—Exercise therapy. |
    Breathing exercises—Therapeutic use. | Qi gong. | BISAC: HEALTH & FITNESS /
    Diseases / Musculoskeletal. | BODY, MIND & SPIRIT / Healing / Energy (Qigong,
    Reiki, Polarity) | HEALTH & FITNESS / Healing.
Classification: LCC: RC933 .Y362 2017 | DDC: 616.7/2206—dc23

Dedicated to my mother,
Madame Yang, Xie-Jin

Romanization of Chinese Words

This book uses the pinyin romanization system of Chinese to English. Pinyin is standard in the People's Republic of China and in several world organizations, including the United Nations. Pinyin, which was introduced in China in the 1950s, replaces the Wade-Giles and Yale systems. In some cases, the more popular spelling of a word may be used for clarity.

Some common conversions:

Pinyin	Also Spelled As	Pronunciation
qi	chi	chē
qigong	chi kung	chē gōng
qin na	chin na	chǐn nǎ
jin	jing	jǐn
gongfu	kung fu	gōng foo
taijiquan	tai chi chuan	tī jē chǔén

For more information, please refer to *The People's Republic of China: Administrative Atlas*, *Reform of the Chinese Written Language*, or a contemporary manual of style.

The author and publisher have taken the liberty of not italicizing words of foreign origin in this text. This decision was made to make the text easier to read. Please see the comprehensive glossary for definitions of Chinese words.

Note from the Publisher

This book, *Pain-Free Joints*, is an abridgement of the larger book by Dr. Yang, Jwing-Ming titled *Arthritis Relief: Chinese Qigong for Healing and Prevention*. This version highlights the exercises you need to treat your arthritis, leaving the richness of qigong's healing history to the preceding fuller edition.

Table of Contents

Foreword

Until the exceptional journey of Marco Polo in the thirteenth century, Europeans viewed scientific, religious, medical, and philosophical ideas in a very limited manner, perceiving themselves as the world's, if not the universe's, center.

Marco Polo brought to Western consciousness but a tiny fraction of long-accumulated Chinese wisdom, including knowledge of the invention of gun powder, the printing press, rocketry, and, of course, the shocking revelation of a huge civilization already thousands of years old.

Had leaders of thirteenth-century Western thought been sufficiently open to new ideas, Marco Polo could have prepared us for a workable medical system based on the Chinese concept of primary energy, a subtle bioelectric force pervading our every cell, common to us all, and capable of preventing illness, healing when ill, and extending life and its quality.

While a great deal of Chinese wisdom was still locked up in the archives of special teachers (masters) under the seal of secrecy, we would nonetheless have learned much about healing from the vast array of material already available in the thirteenth century: acupuncture, herbology, massage, beneficial breathing techniques, and, most importantly, the many ways to manipulate and to increase the flow of this subtle energy force called qi (pronounced *chee*).

Apparently, Western consciousness is at last prepared to receive this grand Chinese legacy, because qigong (energy work) knowledge and training have proliferated in Western society in the last few decades. Western medicine has begun to accept, or at least explore, the existence of qi and its circulation in the body.

Yang, Jwing-Ming, PhD, is indeed a master when describing in numerous published volumes the extensive Chinese concept of qi, explaining not just well-known facets of the lore but also revealing long-hidden secret manuscripts previously unavailable to Western readers.

With the guidance of Dr. Yang, the reader will learn many simple exercises that condition the tissues and permit increased blood flow, and thus oxygen and other nourishment, to those parts of the body in need. More importantly, the reader is taught to "lead" the qi to direct the flow of this primary subtle energy. According to Dr. Yang, "In order to use qigong to maintain and improve your health you must know that there is qi in your body, and you must understand how it circulates and what you can do to ensure that the circulation is smooth and strong." All this, and more, is presented in clear language that flows easily from a very patient teacher. Four thousand years of Chinese observation have resulted in many beneficial methods for preventing illness and achieving wellness, and none are more basic to the arthritic than those described in this book.

Perry A. Chapdelaine Sr. (1925–2015)
Author and past executive director, Arthritis Trust of America

Preface

Arthritis has afflicted humankind for as far back as we can trace. In all races, the young as well as the old have experienced the pain of arthritis. The condition can also have a disastrous effect on the sufferer's peace of mind. Despite the great advances made in many fields of science, Western medicine today is still unable to cure many forms of arthritis. Most treatment is limited to relieving pain and inflammation rather than curing the condition at its root.

In the nearly four thousand years that Chinese medicine has been developing, many approaches have emerged to stopping the pain or even curing arthritis, such as acupuncture, massage, qigong (pronounced *chee gong*) exercises, and herbal treatment.

In this book, I will focus on only the qigong practices commonly used by the Chinese to treat arthritis. Other methods, such as acupuncture and herbal treatments, will have to be introduced elsewhere by qualified Chinese physicians.

Naturally, some methods are more effective than others, depending on the condition of the specific individual. Qigong exercises have come to be considered as an excellent method not only of preventing arthritis, but also of curing many forms of arthritis and rebuilding the strength of the joints. Once the joint completely recovers its strength, it is well on its way to a complete healing.

It is clear that both Western and Eastern medicines have their advantages and disadvantages. If both cultures could share what they have discovered and learn to experience each other with open minds, then medicine would have a chance to begin a new era. Western medicine, for example, would be able to borrow the information that Chinese medicine has accumulated about qi (bioelectricity) and combine it with the findings drawn from its own experience. Chinese medicine, on the other hand, could adapt modern Western medical technology to aid and improve the effectiveness of traditional Oriental medicine.

Arthritis serves as an excellent demonstration of how this combination of Eastern and Western medicine can work. Chinese doctors believe that the main causes of arthritis are weakness and injury of the joints. In order to rebuild the strength of the joints and repair the injury, qi must be led to these joints and be able to circulate smoothly there. Only by nourishing these joints with qi can the damage be repaired. Chinese doctors have researched ways of improving the qi circulation in the joints and have found that the majority of arthritis patients can be healed. In addition, they have found that once the joints are strong again, the arthritis will not readily return.

Since the first edition of this book was published, many people have contacted me about the benefits they have obtained from this book. Many of them could not believe that the serious problem of arthritis can be easily treated by simple exercises. Through acupuncture, massage, or herbal treatment, the relief from arthritis pain is not as long-lasting, yet is also drug-free and promotes a healthier lifestyle. It is also well understood that the long-term solution is through the correct methods of exercises. For example, when an episode is serious, any exercise that can cause tension in the joint area is not proper. This is because the tension of the joint locks the joint, making the qi and blood circulation more stagnant. The key to healing or repairing the joints is through adequate, smooth qi and blood circulation. Only then can the damaged physical areas be rebuilt.

I remember when I was teaching qigong in Andover, Massachusetts, about ten years ago, right after one of my classes there was a senior woman who came to see me for help. She showed me her swollen hands and wrists, caused by a serious arthritis problem. After I took a look, I asked her if she was able to move her fingers and turn her wrists. She tried and showed some ability to move them with limited flexibility. I taught her some simple theory of the importance of circulating the qi and blood in the fingers and wrists. Then, I encouraged her to do the finger and wrist exercises everyday as many times as possible. I also told her it would probably take six months to see the effectiveness of the treatment.

Three months later, she came to see me although I had forgotten about our first meeting and conversation. She showed me her hands, and what I saw were mildly swollen index, middle, and ring fingers. I told her she should be careful, since there was a sign of arthritis development. She stared at me with big eyes and said, "You don't member me, Dr. Yang," and she refreshed my memory of the first meeting. I could not believe it took only three months for her to have this significant progress. She told me she had stopped taking painkillers for nearly a month already. Whenever there was an episode of pain, she simply moved the area for a few minutes and the pain was alleviated.

From this experience, I saw how she had conquered herself in making these activities part of her lifestyle. I also believe that she had grasped the key to healing herself through simple qigong exercises.

Many people think qigong practice is hard and mysterious. In some ways, it is. However, in some other ways, it is simple and effective. Actually, the most difficult task is regulating yourself into practicing as part of your lifestyle. Remember, the most powerful way to maintain health and cure problems is to bring some proper daily exercises and diet into your life. Our physical body is evolved through use and movement. We must keep moving and exercising it. If we ignore this fact, we will degenerate rapidly and become sick easily.

Dr. Yang, Jwing-Ming

How to Use This Book

QIGONG IS A PRACTICE. As you practice the seemingly simple movements you will find the deeper feeling that comes only from practice, and it is this feeling that will lead you to a healthier body. The exercises and massage techniques in chapter 2 will be helpful in alleviating your existing pain and preparing you for the strengthening exercises in chapter 3.

But before you begin you must ask: what, why, and how. "What" means "What am I looking for?" "What do I expect?" and "What should I do?" Then you must ask, "Why do I need it?" "Why does it work?" "Why must I do it this way instead of that way?" Finally, you must ask, "How does it work?" "How much have I advanced toward my goal?" and "How will I be able to advance further?"

It is very important to understand what you are practicing, not just automatically to repeat what you have learned. Understanding is the root of any work. Through understanding you will be able to know your goal. Once you know your goal, your mind can be firm and steady. With this understanding, you will be able to see why something has happened, and what the principles and theories behind it are. Without all of this, your work will be done blindly, and it will be a long and painful process. Only when you are sure what your target is and why you need to reach it should you raise the question of how you are going to accomplish it. The answers to all of these questions form the root of your practice and will help you to avoid the bewilderment and confusion that uncertainty brings. If you keep this root, you will be able to apply the theory and make it grow—you will know how to create. Without this root, what you learn will be only branches and flowers, and in time they will wither.

In China there is a story about an old man who was able to change a piece of rock into gold. One day, a boy came to see him and asked for his help. The old man said, "Boy, what do you want? Gold? I can give you all of the gold you want." The boy replied, "No, master, what I want is not your gold. What I want is the trick of how to change the rock into gold!" When you just have gold, you can spend it all and become poor again. If you have the knowledge of how to make gold, you will never be poor. For the same reason, when you practice, understanding theory and principle will not only shorten your time of pondering and practice but also enable you to practice most efficiently. One of the hardest parts of the training process is learning how actually to do the forms correctly. Every qigong movement has its special meaning and purpose.

CHAPTER 1

What Is Arthritis?

1-1. Introduction

In this chapter, we will first describe arthritis from the point of view of both Western medicine and Chinese medicine. In the next section, we will briefly consider the possible causes of arthritis. Finally, we will review other means of preventing or curing arthritis.

Although both the Western and the Chinese systems of medicine describe arthritis in very similar ways, especially in regard to symptoms, there are a number of differences in how the two cultures approach the disease.

1-2. What Is Arthritis?

Western Viewpoints about Arthritis

Before discussing arthritis, we would first like to mention another popular, nonmedical term, *rheumatism*, which is commonly confused with arthritis. Rheumatism has come to mean so many things to so many people that it is almost impossible to give it a clear definition. The term *rheumatism* commonly refers to any of several pathological conditions of the muscles, tendons, joints, bones, or nerves, characterized by discomfort and disability. This includes variable, shifting, painful inflammation and stiffness of the muscles, joints, or other structures.

The term *arthritis* is also commonly misused to refer to any vague pain in the area of the joints. However, joints are complicated mechanisms made up of ligaments, tendons, muscles, cartilage, and *bursae*, and pain in them can have many different causes. Arthritis is specifically an inflammation of the joints. The word *arthritis* is derived from the Greek words *arthron* (joint) and *itis* (inflammation). Therefore, if you have pain or swelling caused by injury to the ligaments or muscles, it is not necessarily classified as arthritis. You can see that while arthritis is (in a popular sense) a form of rheumatism, rheumatism is not necessarily arthritis.

The symptoms or characteristics of arthritis are pain, swelling, redness, heat, stiffness, and deformity in one or more joints. Arthritis may appear suddenly or gradually, and it may feel different to different people. Some patients feel a sharp, burning, or grinding pain, while others may feel a pain like a toothache. The same person may feel it sometimes as pain and other times as stiffness. If we look more closely at these signs, we can detect certain characteristic physiological changes. These changes include dilation of the blood vessels in the affected area and an increase of blood flow at the site of the inflammation. In addition, there is increased permeability in these vessels, as white blood cells that fight infection infiltrate the diseased tissue. Finally, fluid from the blood can also leak into the tissue and generate edema or swelling. For these reasons, arthritis may affect not only the joints but also other connective tissues of the body. These tissues include several supporting structures, such as muscles, tendons, and ligaments, and the protective coverings of some internal organs.

Chinese Viewpoints about Arthritis

Although the symptoms of arthritis remain the same everywhere, Chinese physicians consider them from a different point of view. Like all other cases of illness, Chinese physicians diagnose by evaluating the imbalance of qi (which the West now calls bioelectricity) in the body, as well as by considering the actual physical symptoms.

Chinese medicine has found that before a physical illness occurs, the qi becomes unbalanced. If this qi imbalance is not corrected, the physical body can be damaged, and the physical symptoms of sickness will appear. The reason for this is very simple. Every cell in your body is alive, and in order to stay alive and functioning, each requires a constant supply of qi. Whenever the supply of qi to the cells becomes irregular (or the qi "loses its balance"), the cells start to malfunction. Chinese physicians try to intercept the problem before there is any actual physical damage and correct the situation with acupuncture, herbal treatments, or a number of other methods. In this way, they hope to prevent physical damage, which is considered the worst stage of an illness. Once the physical body—for example, an internal organ—has been damaged, it is almost impossible to make a complete recovery. This approach is the root of Chinese medicine. Chinese physicians try to diagnose arthritis in its earliest stages, before there is any physical damage. When the qi starts to become unbalanced, although there are no physical changes, the patient suffers from nerve pain. Because human qi is strongly affected by the natural qi present in clouds, moisture, and the sun (both day and night), the body's qi is easily disturbed by changes in the weather, and arthritis patients will usually feel pain in the joints. When cloud cover is low and there is a lot of moisture in the air, the potential of the earth's electromagnetic field is also increased, and your body's qi balance can be significantly influenced. The other obvious symptom of this influence is emotional disturbance. In the West, as long as there is no symptom of physical damage, these feelings of physical and emotional pain are usually ignored, although sometimes drugs are prescribed to stop the pain. Even though Western physicians sometimes consider this an early stage of arthritis, Chinese physicians do not, and refer to it instead as "feng shi," or "wind moisture." This refers to the cause of the pain that the patients feel. Eastern medical dictionaries often translate "feng shi" as "rheumatism."

Although countless arthritis patients regularly feel their pain worsen when the weather changes, scientists who conducted studies in an experimental climate chamber at the University of Pennsylvania concluded that there is no evidence that the weather affects arthritis.[1] I believe that this is solely because Western medicine does not take qi/bioelectricity into account. When Western medicine starts to understand the relationship between environmental qi and human qi, then ample evidence of this association will emerge.

In China, when feng shi occurs, people will usually seek out a physician to correct the problem through acupuncture, massage, acupressure, herbal treatment, qigong exercises, or, most commonly, a combination of these methods. The specific treatment would, of course, depend on the symptoms of each individual case. For example, if the feng shi stems from an old joint injury, the treatment will be different than if it were caused by weak joints. The key to treatment is finding the root of the qi imbalance and correcting it. Only when this root cause is removed will the patient recover completely.

There are many possible causes of feng shi. The most common cause is a joint injury that never completely healed and caused a gradually increasing disturbance of the qi circulation. Fortunately, if the patient practices the correct qigong exercises, the joint can be healed completely and its strength rebuilt. Exercise stimulates the qi and increases its circulation, which removes stagnation and blockages and lets the body's natural healing mechanism operate. Smooth qi circulation is the root of health and the foundation of healing.

Feng shi will frequently also be found in patients who were born with weak joints or deformities, such as having one leg significantly longer than the other. Naturally, the most common and serious cases of feng shi are caused by aging. As we grow older, the muscles and tendons degenerate and start functioning less effectively around the joints, a process that places more pressure on the cartilage, synovium (joint surface), capsule, and the bones. This is the main cause of arthritis in older people.

If a person with feng shi does not seek to correct the problem, or the physician fails to correct it, the feng shi may develop into an infectious joint problem (guan jie yan), which is what the Chinese call arthritis, and the joint will begin to suffer physical damage. The indications of an infectious problem are swelling, redness, pain, stiffness, sometimes fever, and deformity of the joint. This stage is already considered serious. Unlike Western medicine, traditional Chinese medicine does not differentiate among the various forms of arthritis, such as gout and osteoarthritis.

1-3. Causes of Arthritis

Although we understand how some forms of arthritis start, we are still in the dark about other forms. In this section, we would like to summarize the known causes and also contribute some ideas from Chinese medicine and qigong.

Weakness of the Internal Organs

We already know that the condition of the internal organs is closely related to our health. According to Chinese medicine, there are five Yin organs that are considered the most important for our health and longevity. These organs are the heart, liver, lungs, kidneys, and spleen. Whenever any of these five organs is not functioning properly, sickness or even death can occur. Furthermore, all of these five organs are mutually interrelated. Whenever there is a problem with one, the others are always involved too. For example, gouty arthritis is caused by the improper functioning of the liver and kidneys.

Defective Genes

It has been reported that some forms of arthritis are caused by defective genes inherited from one's parents. According to Chinese medicine, genes are considered the essence of your being. This essence is responsible for the production of hormones, from which the production of qi can be enhanced. When this qi is led to the brain, the spirit is raised. When all of these conversion processes are functioning normally, the immune system is strong and sickness is less likely. One of the main goals of qigong is learning how to maintain the production of essence so the qi can be produced efficiently. The abundant qi can then be led to the brain for nourishment.

Weak Joints

Weak joints can come from heredity or from lack of exercise. The body is a living machine, so the more you use it, the better condition it will be in. Chinese medicine believes that even if you have inherited a weak joint, it is still possible to strengthen it through qigong. When you exercise, qi is brought to the joint by the movement of the muscles and tendons. This will nourish the joint and rebuild it.

Injury

According to modern medicine, some forms of arthritis are caused by injury to the joints. Although the injury may not be serious, it may have significant results. The injury can affect the muscles, tendons, ligaments, or even the cartilage and bone. Whenever any joint injury, even a minor one, is not treated, the normal smooth qi circulation in the joint area will be affected. If the situation persists, the qi imbalance can cause problems such as arthritis.

Aging

Aging has always been the cause of many sicknesses, including arthritis. When you are old, the qi level in your body is low. Because your system is being deprived of the required amount of qi, it starts to degenerate. One of the main goals of qigong practice is learning how to slow down the aging process by building up the qi in the body.

Qi Deficiency

Qi deficiency is responsible for many problems. It can be caused by emotional depression and sadness, which can lead the qi inward and make the body yin. This deprives the outer body of qi. When this happens, you will generally feel cold. If the problem persists for a long time, the muscles and tendons will be affected by the lack of qi, and the joints will be weakened.

Qi deficiency can have other causes, such as the weather. For example, your body's qi is more deficient in the winter, and therefore arthritis can be more serious then.

Qi deficiency can also be caused by working for prolonged periods in a damp area or by exposing your joints to the cold.

Tension

Tension includes both mental tension and physical tension, which are related and cannot be separated. Constant mental and physical tension can increase the pressure on the joints. For example, some people are very tense and grind their teeth in their sleep, which can cause arthritis in the jaw.

Most body tension is caused by emotional disturbance, which is related to your mental reaction to stressful events. For this reason, learning how to regulate your mind is an important part of the treatment of arthritis.

1-4. Other Possible Means of Preventing or Curing Arthritis

In addition to those already discussed, there are a number of other methods for preventing or curing arthritis. Although many of them are still awaiting scientific confirmation, they may be worth your consideration. However, you must understand that everybody has his or her own unique characteristics and his or her own unique inheritance. In addition to the habits and lifestyle that each person has developed, everyone's mental and physical structure is different. For example, some people are affected by allergies while others are not. What this means is that you cannot necessarily use the same method to treat different people, even when they have the same disease. Even modern Western medicine has found that the same treatment will not work equally well on all patients. Therefore, do not automatically brush off some of the treatment methods we will discuss. After all, Western medicine is only in its infancy, and it may come to understand and accept these alternative remedies.

Diet

People who are experienced in qigong have always understood food to be a significant influence on the condition of the qi in the body. For this reason, diet is one of the main concerns of Chinese medicine. There is a saying: "You are what you eat." It is well known that improper diet is one of the main causes of gouty arthritis. The Chinese have found many different herbs that can ease the pain and reduce the swelling of arthritis. It has recently been discovered that protein, calories, and fats can reduce the inflammation of arthritis. Certain fish oils may interfere with the process of inflammation and therefore reduce the symptoms of rheumatoid arthritis.[2, 3]

Change of Residence

Because the qi in your environment can affect the qi in your body, arthritis sufferers should give serious consideration to this approach. If the climate where you live is too damp or too cold, it may be affecting your arthritis. It has recently been discovered that the qi in our bodies can be significantly affected by the electromagnetic fields generated by modern technology, and therefore cause some forms of cancer. For example, people who live near high-tension power lines tend to get cancer more often than those who do not. Perhaps similar environmental effects on arthritis will be found.

Change of Lifestyle

Your lifestyle affects how the qi circulates in your body. If you frequently feel ill, especially mentally, you might need to change your lifestyle. How you think and how you coordinate the qi pattern in your body with the natural qi is very important for your health. Whenever your qi circulation is against the "Dao" (nature), you will be sick. You may find that walking for an hour or doing qigong exercises every morning improves your qi circulation.

Clothing

What you wear also affects the qi in your body. In the winter, you must stay warm and especially protect your joints. Joints that are left unprotected can lose qi very quickly.

It has been discovered that many man-made fibers can adversely affect the qi distribution and circulation in the body. For example, polyester is known to cause qi stagnation and to prevent the body's qi from exchanging with the environmental qi. You may have noticed that clothing made of polyester can accumulate a considerable charge of static electricity in the winter. This builds up an electromagnetic field and affects the qi circulation in your body.

There are many other ways to improve the status of your arthritis. For example, it is reported that sexual activity can stimulate the adrenal glands to produce more corticosteroid, a hormone that reduces joint inflammation and pain. It is believed that sexual activity may also trigger the release of endorphins, a naturally occurring pain-killing substance.[4]

You can see from our brief discussion that if we want to understand arthritis completely, we must remain humble and continue our study and research. Only then will we be able to reach the goal of a complete cure.

References

1. Decker, John L., *Medicine for the Layman—Arthritis* (Bethesda, MD: Office of Clinical Reports and Inquiries, National Institutes of Health, 1982).
2. Arthritis Foundation, *Arthritis and Diet* (Atlanta, GA: Arthritis Foundation, n.d.).
3. University of California, Berkeley, "Can Diet Relieve Arthritis?" *Wellness Letter* 6(8).
4. "Arthritis and Your Love Life," *Men's Health* (1989), 8.

CHAPTER 2

How Do the Chinese Treat Arthritis?

2-1. Introduction

In the first chapter, we said that the actual definition of qigong is the study of qi. This means that qigong covers a very wide field of research and includes the study of the three general types of qi (heaven qi, earth qi, and human qi) and their interrelationships. However, because the Chinese have traditionally paid more attention to the study of human qi, which is concerned with health and longevity, the term *qigong* has often been misunderstood and misused to mean only the study of human qi. Because so much attention has been given to human qi over thousands of years, the study of human qigong has reached a very high level. Today, it includes many fields such as acupuncture, herbal study, massage, cavity press, qigong exercises, and even martial arts.

In this chapter, I would like to summarize, according to my understanding, some of the methods commonly used in China to prevent arthritis, to ease its pain, and to cure it. I would then like to focus the discussion on how qigong uses massage (including cavity press) and exercises to prevent and cure arthritis. Finally, I would like to point out the differences in how Western and Chinese medicine use massage and exercise to treat arthritis.

2-2. General Chinese Treatments for Arthritis

The best way to treat arthritis is to prevent it from happening. However, if it has already occurred, then the appropriate course is to prevent it from getting any worse, and then to rebuild the strength of the joint so that it can resume functioning normally.

Generally speaking, if a case of arthritis has already reached the stage of serious physical damage, special treatment is needed before any rebuilding can proceed. During the treating and rebuilding process, alleviating pain is always the first concern. In this section, we will briefly discuss the theory behind several common methods for treating arthritis that have been developed in China.

Massage

When done properly, massage will improve the qi circulation in the joint area. Massage is commonly used when a patient suffers from feng shi before arthritis and physical damage have occurred. At this time, the qi circulation is unbalanced, which may affect the nerves around the joints and cause pain. As mentioned earlier, feng shi can occur when a joint is weak or injured, or when a joint has degenerated because of aging. The pain usually increases when rain is coming on, because clouds and moisture accumulate great masses of electric charges that affect the qi in our bodies. Pain can also occur when the joints are exposed to cold wind, which can significantly affect the qi of the joints.

If the feng shi is caused by a minor injury, massage can help to heal the injury and ease the pain. The massage can usually prevent the feng shi from developing into arthritis, which the Chinese call "joint infection" (guan jie yan). However, if the feng shi is caused by a weak joint or one degenerated because of aging, then once the pain is alleviated, qigong exercises are necessary to rebuild the strength of the joint and prevent the feng shi from returning and developing into arthritis.

Massage can be used to heal feng shi, and it is very effective in increasing qi circulation and easing the pain even when the joint infection (arthritis) has already become serious. However, because massage cannot reach deep enough into the body, it is not wise to rely on it for a cure.

Acupuncture

Acupuncture is another method of temporarily stopping the pain and can increase the qi circulation in the joint area to help in its healing. The main difference between massage and acupuncture is that the former usually stays only on the surface, while the latter can reach to the center of the joint. One of the advantages of acupuncture is that if the arthritis is caused by an old injury deep in the joint, it can heal the injury or at least remove some of the stagnated qi or bruise.

In acupuncture, needles or other newly developed means such as lasers or electricity are used to stimulate and increase the qi circulation. Although acupuncture can stop the pain and can, to some degree, cure the arthritis, the process can be so time-consuming as to be emotionally draining. Acupuncture is an external method, and while it may remove the symptoms, it can usually heal arthritis only temporarily or only to a limited degree. Rebuilding the strength of the joint is a long-term proposition. Therefore, after arthritis patients have received some treatment, the physician will frequently encourage them to get involved in qigong exercises to rebuild the joint.

Herbal Treatments

Herbal treatments are used together with massage and acupuncture, especially when the arthritis is caused by an injury. The herbs are usually made into a paste or ground into powder, mixed with a liquid such as alcohol, and then applied to the joint. The dressing is changed every twenty-four hours.

Herbal treatments are used to alleviate pain, to increase the qi circulation and help the healing of the injury, and to speed up the process of regrowth. Patients who work to rebuild weak joints through qigong exercises can speed the process with herbal treatments.

Cavity Press

Cavity press (dian xue) is the method of using the fingertips (especially the thumb tip) to press acupuncture cavities and certain other points (pressure points) on the body in order to manipulate the qi circulation. Acupuncture cavities are tiny spots distributed over the entire body where the qi of the body can be manipulated through massage or the insertion of needles. According to our new understanding of bioelectricity, these cavities are places where the electrical conductivity is higher than in neighboring areas. They are therefore more sensitive to external stimulation, and they allow this external stimulation to reach to the primary qi channels.[1] Strictly speaking, cavity press (acupressure) should be discussed under massage. However, its theory is deeper and somewhat different from general massage. General massage covers a larger area of the joint, while cavity press focuses on the acupuncture cavities and certain non-acupuncture points. Normally, the power in cavity press can reach much deeper than in general massage. Furthermore, cavity press mostly uses the qi channels to improve qi circulation inside the joint, while general massage can enhance qi circulation only superficially.

The theory of cavity press is very similar to that of acupuncture. There are a few differences, however: (a) acupuncture uses needles or other means of penetration such as lasers, while cavity press uses the fingertips to press the cavities; (b) acupuncture can reach much deeper than cavity press; (c) cavity press is easier and more convenient than acupuncture, which requires equipment and a higher level of training; and (d) a patient can use cavity press on himself or herself much more easily than acupuncture. Anyone can learn to use cavity press to treat arthritis after only a short period of training and some experience. However, it takes years of study to learn acupuncture.

In cavity press, stagnant qi deep in the joint is led to the surface. This improves the qi circulation in the joint area and reduces the pain considerably. The use of cavity press to speed up the healing of injured joints is very common in Chinese martial arts.

Qigong Exercises

The main purpose of qigong exercises for arthritis is to rebuild the strength of the joint by improving the qi circulation. As mentioned earlier, traditional Chinese physicians believe that because the body's cells are alive, as long as there is a proper supply of qi, the physical damage can be repaired or even completely rebuilt. They have proven that broken bones can be mended completely, even in the elderly. Even some Western physicians have now come to believe that damaged or degenerated joints can be returned to their original healthy state.[2]

Practicing qigong can not only heal arthritis or joint injury and rebuild the joint, but it is also known to be very effective in strengthening the internal organs. Many illnesses, including some forms of arthritis, stem from abnormally functioning internal organs. For example, gouty arthritis is caused by an improperly functioning liver and kidneys.[3] According to Chinese medicine, almost all illnesses are caused by abnormal qi circulation. Internal organs are the devices that produce and manage the circulation of qi. Keeping organs healthy is the key to health and longevity, and qigong is one of the most effective ways of doing so. Chinese physicians also believe that when the internal organs are healthy, the immune system will be healthy, and the potential for resisting sickness will be high. A weak immune system is responsible for many illnesses, and is considered to be closely related to the occurrence of arthritis. For example, lupus erythematosus, rheumatoid arthritis, Lyme disease, Sjögren's syndrome, and scleroderma are all linked to a weak immune system.[3,4]

Before we discuss massage and qigong exercises, let us get an overview of the differences in how Chinese and Western medicine treat arthritis.

Western and Eastern Approaches to Treating Arthritis: An Overview

1. Prevention

Western medicine: There are few documents that discuss how to prevent arthritis. It just does not seem to be considered important. Only when the symptoms of arthritis appear is treatment started. Even if there is some joint pain and if there is no sign of arthritis in the X-rays, the physician may prescribe some medication for the pain, but other than that, he or she will all too often tend to ignore it.

Chinese medicine: When a patient has a joint injury, Chinese physicians will first usually use acupuncture, massage, and herbal treatment to eliminate any bruises or qi stagnation inside the joint. When the injury is almost healed, the physician will encourage the patient to do qigong exercises to increase the qi circulation and speed up the healing. The most important effect of the qigong, however, is to ensure that all the bruises and stagnation in the joint are cleared up. This can be done only through the patient moving the joint. If this is not done, the bruises and stagnation will eventually develop into feng shi and continue to interfere with smooth and balanced qi circulation in the joint.

In China, when people start getting older and feel their bodies getting weaker, they will often start practicing some form of qigong such as taijiquan or Ba Duan Jin (Eight Pieces of Brocade).[5,6] The practice helps them to keep their qi circulating smoothly and to slow down the degeneration of their bodies. It also prevents feng shi and arthritis. Most people find that in addition to strengthening their limbs, they are also able to restore their internal organs to full health, which is the key to health and longevity.

2. Stopping the pain

Western medicine: Western medicine sometimes uses massage to alleviate pain, but more commonly, drugs such as aspirin, prednisone, naproxen, ibuprofen, colchicine, and many others are prescribed. The problem with drugs is that very often, they have side effects, such as the disturbance of the gastrointestinal tract and skin rash caused by using ibuprofen, and the weakening or damaging of the internal organs caused by other medicines.[1] This is a very common problem in Western medicine, which will frequently cure one problem only to inflict another one on the patient.

Chinese medicine: Acupuncture, massage, cavity press, and herbal treatments are commonly used to stop the pain. The treatments are used only to make the patient feel more comfortable and are not considered part of the healing.

3. Healing

Western medicine: Drugs can be effective in treating some forms of arthritis. For example, certain drugs can be used to regulate the liver and the kidneys, curing gouty arthritis. This approach can get quick results. However, the patient is then reliant on the drugs, which may eventually disturb the normal functioning of some organs.

When the arthritis has become serious, the joint can now be replaced with an artificial one. However, the long-term effect of these replacement joints is still unknown.[3,4] Doctors now encourage arthritis patients to do certain exercises, often with significant results. However, documentation and more experimentation are still needed. For example, are there some forms of exercise that are harmful rather than beneficial to arthritis patients? So far, there is no established authority on this subject.

Electricity is now being used to speed up the healing of broken bones. As the West increases its understanding of bioelectricity (qi), it is quite possible that ways will be found to use electricity to speed up the healing and regrowth of arthritic joints.

Chinese medicine: Massage, cavity press, and acupuncture are usually used first to increase the qi circulation. If the arthritis is not too serious, these methods may be sufficient for a cure. However, if the arthritis has become serious, external and internal herbal treatments are also called for. The herbs taken internally help to increase the qi circulation, remove bruises, or prevent further infection of the joint. Chinese medicine seeks to cure the cause of the arthritis. For example, if it is caused by an injury, then bruises and qi stagnation must be cleared up. And if the arthritis is caused by degeneration due to aging, then qigong exercises must be used to rebuild the joint and slow the degeneration.

In the next section, we will discuss in more detail how massage and qigong exercises can prevent and cure arthritis.

2-3. How Does Qigong Cure Arthritis?

In Chinese medicine, the concept of qi is used both during diagnosis and during treatment. A basic principle of Chinese medicine is that you must rebalance the qi before you can cure the root of a disease. Only then can you also repair the physical damage and rebuild your physical strength and health. The theory is very simple. Your entire body is made up of living cells. When these cells receive the proper qi supply, they will function normally and even repair themselves. However, if the qi supply is abnormal, and this condition persists, then even though the cells were originally healthy, they will be damaged or changed (perhaps even becoming cancerous). In light of this basic qi theory, let us first discuss why qigong can be effective in curing arthritis. Then we will explain how Chinese massage and qigong work, and finally we will point out the main differences in how Western and Chinese medicine use massage and exercise to treat arthritis.

Why Qigong Is Effective for Arthritis

1. Qigong maintains and increases smooth qi circulation

As mentioned earlier, the goal of qigong healing is to reestablish a strong, smooth flow of qi through the affected area. When this happens, the physical damage can be repaired and the strength rebuilt. Chinese physicians have always believed that as long as you are alive, physical damage to the body can be repaired through improving the qi and blood circulation. Most Western physicians do not agree but believe that the osteoarthritis caused by aging and the degeneration of the joints cannot be reversed. However, some Western physicians have changed their minds about this.[2]

2. Qigong strengthens the organs

The greatest benefit of Chinese qigong most likely lies in the training that is designed to regulate the qi circulating in the internal organs. We know that these organs are vital, and if there is any problem with them, we can become sick or even die. Regulating their qi and keeping them healthy is a major goal of qigong. In the more advanced qigong practices, the training goes even deeper and is concerned with strengthening and improving the health of the organs. These practices balance the yin and yang qi in the organs to slow down the aging process. Because the internal organs manage the various functions of your body, you must take care of them first if you want to slow down the aging process.

The qi circulating in your body is the source of your life. When this circulation stops, you die. Let us look again at the source or origin of your qi. Qi is energy, and it has to be produced from matter. As explained in the first chapter, the Chinese believe that the body contains two types of material that can be converted into qi: one is called prebirth essence and the other postbirth essence. The prebirth essence is inherited from your parents, while the postbirth essence is in the food and the air you take in after your birth. Only in this century was it discovered that prebirth essence is actually the hormones produced by the endocrine glands. Because the quality and quantity of the hormones you produce depend on the inherent strength of your body, determined by the genes you received from your parents, qigong practitioners believe that the genes were the prebirth essence.

The formation of your organs is controlled by your genes. Once you are born, your organs are significantly affected by your lifestyle, which includes your thinking (emotional disturbances), food, air, and even the weather you are exposed to. Your internal organs convert food and air into the qi that circulates in your body. Any trouble in the internal organs will affect the production of qi. Remember, only when your internal organs are healthy will you have a normal supply of qi, and only then will you be able to manage your life efficiently.

Your qi can be affected by defects in your organs. The physical body is closely related to the qi, and they affect each other. Whenever the qi loses balance, its manifestation in the physical body will be abnormal. We know today that many diseases not confined to the organs are caused by the abnormal functioning of the organs. You can see that the condition of the internal organs is actually the foundation of your health and longevity.

3. Qigong strengthens the immune and hormone-production systems

Western science knows that the body's immune system is closely related to the endocrine glands, which produce hormones. Hormones, as they are now understood, do not actually create processes. What they do, however, is cause fundamental processes such as growth and reproduction to speed up or slow down. (The word *hormone* comes from the Greek word *hormikz*, which means "to excite, to stimulate, or to stir up.") They also strengthen the ability of the immune system to fight diseases. For example, it is believed that the thymus gland (which is located just behind the top of the sternum) plays an important role in the body's immune system. Exactly how this happens is still not completely understood. We also do not know very much about the pineal gland in the upper back part of the brain, nor do we have a full understanding of the function of the thymus.[7] In fact, it has only recently come to be believed that hormone production is significantly related to the aging process.

Many of us know of people who were deathly sick, but who had a very high spirit and a strong desire to survive, and miraculously recovered. Both Western and Eastern religions tell of many such cases. Chinese qigong practitioners believe that if a sick person can lead qi to the brain through concentration or through a strong desire, he or she can evoke a powerful healing force. A possible explanation is that the stronger qi flow activates the pineal and pituitary glands so that they generate more hormones. We now know that the most important function of the pituitary gland is to stimulate, regulate, and coordinate the functions of the other endocrine glands.[7] For this reason, it is sometimes called the "master gland."

In Chinese qigong, the upper dan tian (shang dan tian, center of brain) is considered the center of your whole being. If you raise your spirit, which resides there, you can energize your body, generate amazing physical and mental strength, and recover more quickly from injury or sickness. Certain groups in the West have also recognized its importance as the center of the spirit—through the "third eye," one is able to sense further than the physical eyes can see.

If we combine the understanding of old and new, East and West, we can conclude that what actually happens, probably because of mental concentration, is that a stronger current of bioelectricity is led to the pineal and pituitary glands to activate the production of hormones. This stimulates the entire endocrine system and causes it to function more effectively, improving healing, reproduction, and growth. If this is correct, then it is possible to begin a new era of scientific self-healing or spiritual healing. An alternative result is that we may learn how to devise electrical equipment to activate the pineal and pituitary glands to improve the effectiveness and speed of healing. Perhaps we may also be able to find the secret key to slowing down the aging process.

4. Qigong raises the spirit of vitality

The spirit is closely tied to the mind and cannot be separated from it. In qigong practice, the mind is considered the general in the battle against sickness. When the mind (general) has a strong will, thoroughly understands the battlefield (the body), wisely and carefully sets up the strategy (the breathing technique), and effectively and efficiently manages the soldiers (the qi), then the morale (spirit) of the general and soldiers can be high. When this happens, sickness can be conquered and health regained.

When you use qigong to treat your arthritis, you must first treat your mind by changing the way you look at your sickness and your life. The first thing you need to do is to stop passively accepting the negative things that have happened to you. Become more active and take charge of your life. Most basically, learn how to keep the pain of arthritis from disturbing your peace of mind. Remember, doing something is better than doing nothing.

Second, you must rebuild your confidence in your ability to treat your arthritis. Even though you may have failed before, don't let that discourage you. Learn about the causes of your problem, understand the theory of this new treatment, and try to think about how you can make the treatment more effective. Once you have done this, you will have rebuilt your confidence not only in the treatment but also in your life.

Once you have built up your confidence, the third thing you need to do is to develop the willpower, patience, and perseverance needed to keep up the treatment. The best way to prevent the arthritis from returning once you have cured it is to make qigong part of your life.

Fourth, after you have practiced qigong for a while, you will understand your body better and you will know how to deal with the problems more easily. You may realize that the pain is not necessarily all bad. Pain draws your attention to your body and helps you to understand yourself better. Pain can also help you to build up willpower and perseverance. However, you must first know what pain is; only then will you know how to stop it. This is called regulating your mind. Remember that medication is only a temporary solution.

You can see that Chinese qigong heals by going to the root of the problem. It improves the entire body, both mentally and physically, and strengthens the immune system. Only when this is accomplished will the illness be healed completely. Now that you understand why qigong can cure arthritis, let us discuss how qigong reaches this goal.

How Can Qigong Exercises Cure Arthritis, and How Are They Different from Western Arthritis Exercises?

You probably already know that Western physicians recommend exercise for arthritis, and that many books and reports of experiments have been published.[8-13] Regardless of whether you are familiar with these exercises, you should first understand the differences between the exercises used by Chinese qigong and the exercises recommended by Western arthritis physicians. Then your mind will be clear, and you will be able to practice effectively.

First let us review the basic theory of the arthritis exercises used in the West that have proven effective. Naturally, there is no doubt that many of these theories, and even some of the practices, are consistent with those of Chinese qigong.

According to the Western conception, the key to healing arthritis is that the patient must learn how to balance exercise and rest. This means that without exercise there is no hope of healing, but too much exercise will worsen the arthritic condition. Therefore, because each individual has specific arthritic conditions, he or she must first understand the condition and then use common sense to regulate his or her lifestyle and exercise.

Western medicine believes that exercise has several benefits for the physical body: it increases the strength and flexibility of the muscles and ligaments surrounding the joints; it maintains or increases bone strength; and some active types of exercises such as long-distance walking and swimming have important effects on the heart that can promote increased endurance and circulation and fight deterioration of the arteries. It is believed that even a small amount of exercise will help the patient overcome fatigue.

The basic Western theory of how exercise is able to heal arthritis is very simple. Every tissue in your body requires nutrition to work normally and effectively, and most tissues have arteries to carry nutrients to them. However, the situation is quite different for the joint cartilage. In the joints, movement is the only way nourishment can be brought by the synovial fluid to the cartilage and waste products can be removed. This means that exercise promotes good joint nutrition.

According to their different purposes, there are three general types of exercise recommended by Western physicians. The first type is stretching. Usually, this type of exercise is designed to maintain and improve joint mobility, and consequently it decreases pain and improves function. In this type of exercise, the joint is moved or stretched as far as it will comfortably go and then pushed a little further to just past the point where pain or discomfort begins.

The second type of exercise is to increase muscle strength and consequently lend stability to vulnerable joints. However, the exercises designed for this purpose should minimize stress on the joints to avoid further injury. Therefore, many of these exercises are designed to extend and contract the muscles without moving the joints. An example of this is squeezing the fists tight and then relaxing them.

When the joint has partially recovered, the third type of exercise ensures that it stays healthy. This is accomplished through endurance exercises such as walking, swimming, bicycling, jogging, or dancing to promote cardiovascular fitness. An ideal arthritis exercise program should include all three types.

You can see from this review how Western arthritis exercises are able to treat arthritis. What, then, are the differences between them and Chinese qigong?

1. From the theoretical point of view, qigong originates from the concept of regulating the qi (from an imbalanced condition

into a balanced one) both before and after any physical damage has occurred. Western medicine, however, does not yet fully accept the existence of qi or bioelectricity, and is therefore not concerned with it.

2. Chinese qigong considers the regulation of the body to be the most basic and important factor in successful practice. Regulating the body means to bring your body into a very relaxed, centered, and balanced state. Only then can your mind be calm and comfortable. When the body is relaxed, the qi can circulate freely and be led easily anywhere you wish, such as to the skin or even deep into the bone marrow and the internal organs. To cure arthritis, you have to be so relaxed that you can lead the qi deep into the joint where it can repair the damage. Western arthritis exercises are not usually specifically concerned with relaxation.

The first priority in qigong exercises for arthritis is learning how to relax and avoid muscle/tendon tension and stress in the joint area, which is especially critical in severe cases of arthritis. Chinese physicians reason that exercises that tense the muscles and tendons will inhibit the qi circulation from going deep into the damaged joint. Furthermore, tension of the muscles and tendons increases pressure on the joint and can increase the damage. Therefore, Chinese physicians recommend relaxed, gentle movements first to smoothly increase the qi circulation. Only when the patient has rebuilt the strength of the joint will the muscles and tendons be exercised. After all, strong muscles and tendons are what will prevent future joint damage.

3. With qigong, in addition to the body being relaxed, the breathing must be long, deep, and calm. According to qigong theory, breathing is the strategic part of your practice. When you exhale, you instinctively and naturally lead qi to the surface of your body, and when you inhale, you lead it inward to the bone

marrow and the internal organs. In qigong, you have to learn to breathe deeply and calmly in coordination with your thinking. This way, your mind can lead the qi strongly into the damaged area. In Western arthritis exercises, only a few reports even mention breathing.[8]

4. The mind is one of the major forces (EMF, electromotive force) of qi or bioelectric circulation; it has an important role in healing. In order to make your qigong practice really effective, and in addition to regulating your body and breathing, you must also regulate your mind. Regulating your mind means to lead it away from outside distractions and turn it toward feeling what is going on inside your body. In order to lead qi to the damaged places in your body, your mind must be calm, relaxed, and concentrated so that you can feel or sense the qi. The mind, therefore, plays a very important role in qigong. Western arthritis exercises, on the other hand, are usually not concerned with the mind at all.

5. Another significant difference between qigong and Western arthritis exercises is that qigong emphasizes not only healing the joints but also rebuilding the health of the internal organs. Remember, only when the internal organs are healthy can the root of the qi imbalance be removed and, therefore, the cause of the sickness be corrected. Qigong is concerned with bringing the organs back to a healthy state, and it also works to strengthen them. The Western arthritis exercises, in contrast, are not at all concerned with the health of the internal organs.

6. One of the most significant results of qigong practice is maintaining hormone production at a healthy level, which keeps the immune system functioning effectively. In Western medicine, imbalanced hormone production is adjusted with drugs.

7. The most significant difference between qigong and Western arthritis exercise is probably that practicing qigong draws the

patient gradually into an acquaintance with the inner energy of his or her body. Once this is experienced, patients can start to feel energy imbalances when they are just beginning and consequently are able to correct them before physical damage occurs. In fact, this is the key to preventing most illnesses.

Although many of the movements of qigong and Western arthritis exercises are similar, the theory of qigong is more profound, and therefore the challenge is more significant. In fact, the best way to maintain your health and rebuild your qi and body is by understanding the theory of qigong and starting the training.

Because this book will also introduce qigong massage for arthritis, we would like to point out some of the major differences between qigong massage and regular Western massage.

How Chinese Qigong Massage Differs from Western Massage

1. Chinese massage pays attention to improving the circulation of both qi and blood, while Western massage normally emphasizes only good blood circulation and a comfortable, easy feeling.

2. In Chinese massage, the massager and the patient must communicate with each other both through touch and through deeper levels of contact. This mutual cooperation enables the massager to use his or her mind to either lead qi into the patient or to remove excess qi from the patient's body. Therefore, qigong massage requires a higher level of experience and training in concentration. This means that the massage is not limited to only a physical massage; it is also a qi massage. The most important part of this cooperation is that the patient can use his or her own mind to relax the area being massaged and make the massage more effective. Furthermore, this coopera-

tion helps the patient to calm the mind and relax deeply into the internal organs and bone marrow, which makes it possible for the massage to regulate the qi. In Western massage, the coordination between the massager and the patient is not emphasized.

3. Cavity press or acupressure techniques are considered qigong massage. Like Japanese shiatsu massage, which is derived from Chinese acupressure, finger pressure on the cavities is used to regulate the qi circulation and to remove qi and blood stagnation in the affected areas. To do this kind of massage effectively requires not only that the massager knows the location of the cavities, but that he or she also understands the twelve qi channels and how to use them to remove excess qi from affected areas and bring in nourishing qi. It is also extremely helpful if the massager is experienced in qigong. This kind of practice is almost completely ignored in Western massage.

With a bit of practice, you can learn how to use massage to regulate the qi. All you really need to know is the location of the cavities or pressure points around the afflicted joint and how to apply pressure with your finger. After you have gained some experience, you may even wish to study qigong massage and learn more about using it for healing. In this book we will focus only on the massage and cavity press techniques that are related to arthritis. If you are interested in pursuing the subject in more depth, read my book *Qigong Massage: Fundamental Techniques for Health and Relaxation*.

References

1. Robert O. Becker and Gary Selden, *The Body Electric* (New York: William Morrow, 1985).
2. Gifford-Jones, "Keeping the Human Body Active Reduces Risk of Osteoarthritis," *Globe and Mail*, January 31, 1989.

3. John L. Decker, *Medicine for the Layman—Arthritis* (Bethesda, MD: Clinical Center Office of Clinical Reports & Inquiries, 1983).

4. "An Overview of Arthritis and Related Disorders," *Caring*, January 1989.

5. Yang, Jwing-Ming, *Tai Chi Qigong* (Wolfeboro, NH: YMAA Publication Center, 2013).

6. Yang, Jwing-Ming, *Simple Qigong Exercises for Health* (Wolfeboro, NH: YMAA Publication Center, 2013).

7. Benjamin F. Miller, *The Complete Medical Guide* (New York: Simon & Schuster, 1978).

8. Kate Lorig and James F. Fries, "Use It or Lose It," *Aim Plus*, January/February, 1989.

9. Peggy Person, "The Good News about Exercises," *Arthritis Today*, May/June, 1989.

10. "How to Choose the Right Exercise," *Arthritis Today*, January/February, 1987.

11. Irving Kushner, *Understanding Arthritis* (New York: Scribner, 1984).

12. Richard S. Panush and David G. Brown, "Exercise and Arthritis," *Sports Medicine* 4 (1987): 54–64.

13. Fred L. Savage, *Osteo-Arthritis* (Barrytown, NY: Station Hill Press, 1988).

CHAPTER 3

Qigong for Arthritis

3-1. Introduction

In this section, we will introduce some simple stretching techniques, exercises, and massage techniques that can be used to improve and even heal the condition of your joints. These are techniques I have found to be effective over many years of experience. We will first present exercises to strengthen and maintain the health of the internal organs, then consider massage and cavity press techniques, and finally exercises to rebuild the strength of the joints.

Before proceeding any further, we would like to discuss the attitude you need to adopt in your practice. Quite frequently, people who are ill are reluctant to become involved in the healing process. This is especially true for arthritis patients. Both Western and Chinese physicians have had difficulty persuading them to become involved in regular exercise or qigong. The main reason for this reluctance is that the patients are afraid of pain and therefore believe that these kinds of exercise are harmful. In order to conquer this obstacle to your healing, you must understand the theory of healing and the reason for practicing. Only then will you have the confidence necessary for continued practice. Remember, a physician may have an excellent prescription for your illness, but if you don't take the medicine, it won't do you any good.

Another factor that has caused the failure of many a potential cure is lack of persistence. Because the healing process is very slow, it is easy to become impatient and lazy. Often in life, we will know exactly what it is we need to do, but because we are controlled by the emotional parts of our minds, we end up either not doing what we need to or not doing it correctly.

It seems that most of the time our "emotional mind" and "wisdom mind" are in opposition. In China there is a proverb: "You are your own biggest enemy." This means that your emotional mind often wants to go in the opposite direction from what your wisdom mind knows is best. If your wisdom mind is able to overcome your emotional mind, then there is nothing that can stop you from doing anything you want. Usually, however, your emotional mind causes you to lose your willpower and perseverance. We always know that our clear-headed wisdom mind understands what needs to be done, but too often we surrender to our emotional mind and become slaves of our emotions.

The first step when you decide to practice qigong is to strengthen your wisdom mind and use it to govern your emotional mind. Only then will you have enough patience and perseverance to keep practicing. You can see that the first key to successful training is not the techniques themselves but rather your self-control. I sincerely believe that as long as you have a strong will, patience, and perseverance, there is nothing you can't accomplish.

Forming the habit of practicing regularly actually represents changing your lifestyle. Once you have started regulating your life through qigong, not only can it cure your arthritis and restrengthen your joints, but it can also keep you healthy and make both your mental and physical lives much happier.

This chapter will focus on discussing the qigong practices I am familiar with, leaving other methods such as acupuncture and herbs to other references. Before we discuss the actual practices, we would first like to remind you of the keys to successful practice. Only if you follow these keys in your practice will you be able to see and feel how Chinese qigong is different from similar Western arthritis exercises.

Important Training Keys

1. Regulating the Body

Before you start your qigong exercises, you should first calm down your mind and use this mind to bring your body into a calm and relaxed state. Naturally, you should always be concerned with your mental and physical centers. Only then will you be able to find your balance. When you have achieved both mental and physical relaxation, centering, and balance, you will be both natural and comfortable. This is the key to regulating your body.

When you relax, you should learn to relax deeply into your internal organs, and especially the muscles that enclose the organs. In addition, you must also place your mind on the joints that are giving you trouble. The more you can bring your mind deep into the joint and relax it, the more qi will circulate smoothly and freely to repair the damage.

2. Regulating the Breathing

As mentioned before, breathing is the central strategy in qigong practice. According to qigong theory, when you inhale, you lead qi inward and when you exhale you lead qi outward. This is our natural instinct. For example, when you feel cold in the wintertime, in order to keep from letting the qi out of your body, you naturally inhale more than you exhale to lead the qi inward, which also closes the pores in the skin. However, in the summertime when you are too hot, you naturally exhale more than inhale in order to lead qi out of your body. When you do this you start to sweat and the pores open.

In qigong, you want to lead the qi to the internal organs and bone marrow, so you must learn how to use inhalation to lead the qi inward. When you use qigong to cure your arthritis, you must inhale and exhale deeply and calmly so that you can lead the qi deep into the joint and also outward to dissipate the excess or stagnant qi that has accumulated in the joints. Therefore, in addition to relaxing when you practice, you should always remember to inhale and exhale deeply. When you inhale, place your mind deep in the joint, and when you exhale, lead the qi to the surface of the skin.

3. Regulating the Mind

In qigong, the mind is considered the general who directs the battle against sickness. After all, it is your mind that manages all of your thinking and activity. Therefore, a clear, calm mind is very important so that you can judge clearly and accurately. In addition, your attention must also be concentrated. Your mind can generate an EMF (electromotive force or "voltage") that causes your qi to circulate. The more you concentrate, the more strongly you can lead the qi.

When you have a calm and concentrated mind, you will be able to feel and sense the problem correctly. Therefore, when you practice qigong for your arthritis, you must learn how to bring your mind inward so that you can understand the situation, and you must know how to use your concentrated attention to lead the qi.

4. Regulating the Qi

Once you have regulated your body, breathing, and mind, you will be in a good position to start regulating your qi and will be able to lead your qi anywhere in your body in order to make repairs.

5. Regulating the Spirit

The final key to qigong is raising your spirit of vitality. Good morale or fighting spirit is necessary to win the struggle against illness. When your spirit is high, your willpower is strong, your mind is firm, and your patience can last a long time. In addition, when your spirit is high your emotions are under control and your wisdom mind can stimulate the qi to circulate in the body more efficiently. This will significantly reduce the time of healing.

You should now have a clear idea of how to practice most efficiently. During the course of your practice, you should frequently remind yourself of these key requirements. If you would like to learn more about the keys to qigong practice, you may refer to the YMAA book *The Root of Chinese Qigong*.

3-2. Qigong for Strengthening the Internal Organs

Your internal organs are the foundation of your health. Most deaths are due to the malfunction or failure of the internal organs. In order to be healthy and avoid degeneration, your organs need to have the correct amount of qi circulating smoothly through them.

The internal organs manage the energy in our bodies and carry out a variety of physical processes. When any organ starts to malfunction, the qi circulation in the body will be disrupted, and the production of hormones will be affected. This state can result in a variety of disorders, including gouty arthritis.

In this section, we would like to introduce two types of qigong practices that are commonly used to improve qi circulation, especially around the internal organs. The first exercise is massaging the internal organs by moving the muscles inside the torso. If you would like to have more information on the theory behind this subject, please refer to my book *Simple Qigong Exercises for Health*.

The second type of qigong practice is improving the qi circulation around the internal organs by massaging either directly over the organs or on acupuncture cavities that are connected to the organs. If you are interested to know about massage, please refer to my book *Qigong Massage*.

Massaging the Internal Organs with Movement

All of the internal organs are surrounded by muscles. Except for some of the trunk muscles that we use constantly throughout the day, most of these muscles are ignored. According to qigong theory, if you can bring your yi (wisdom mind) to a muscle, you can lead qi to energize it and move it. For example, if you decide you want to be able to wiggle your ears and you keep trying, you will eventually be able to. It's the same with the internal muscles. When you practice becoming very calm and bringing your attention deeper and deeper into the center of your body, you will soon be able to feel and sense the structure and condition of the insides of your body. Once this happens, you can use your mind to move the internal muscles and massage the internal organs.

The way to reach this goal is to start by using your trunk muscles to make the muscles deeper inside your body move. After you have practiced for a while, your mind will be able to reach deeper and feel other muscles as well. Once you are able to feel these muscles, you will be able to move them. With a bit more practice you will be able to control them while keeping them relaxed, and the movements will become natural, easy, and comfortable. Remember that the muscles have to be relaxed before the organs can be relaxed and before the qi can circulate smoothly.

In this subsection, we will introduce the beginning steps of internal organ massage through trunk movement. After you are able to do these exercises easily and smoothly, you should continue to lead your mind deeper and deeper into your body and sense your organs.

It is a good idea to loosen up your trunk before starting these massaging movements. This will let you move more naturally and comfortably.

Loosening the Torso Muscles

The torso is the center of the whole body, and it contains the muscles that control the torso and also surround the internal organs. When the torso muscles are tense, the whole body will be tense and the internal organs will be compressed. This causes stagnation of the qi circulation in the body and especially in the organs. For this reason, the torso muscles should be stretched and loosened up before any moving qigong practice.

The torso is supported by the spine and the trunk muscles. Once you have stretched your trunk muscles, you can loosen up the torso. This also moves the muscles inside your body around, which moves and relaxes your internal organs. This, in turn, makes it possible for the qi to circulate smoothly inside your body.

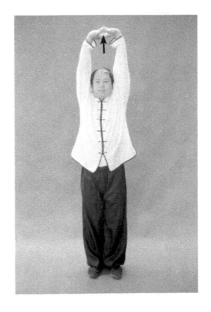

■ Interlock your fingers and lift your hands up over your head, rotating the palms to face upward, while imagining that you are pushing upward with your hands and pushing downward with your feet. Do not tense your muscles, because this will constrict your body and prevent you from stretching. If you do this stretch correctly, you will feel the muscles in your waist area tensing slightly because they are being pulled simultaneously from the top and the bottom. Next, use your mind to relax even more, and stretch out a little bit more. Stretch for about ten seconds.

- After you have stretched for about ten seconds, turn your upper body to one side to twist the trunk muscles. Stay to the side for three to five seconds, then turn your body to face forward and then turn to the other side. Stay there for three to five seconds. Repeat the upper body twisting three times to each side.

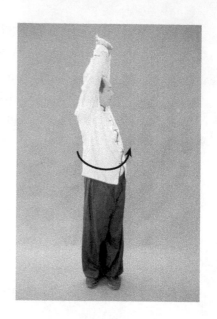

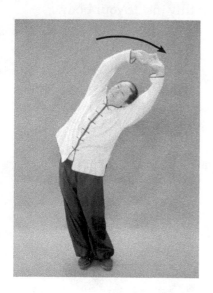

- Next, tilt your upper body to the side and stay there for about three seconds, then tilt to the other side. Tilt three times to each side.

- Next, bend forward and touch your hands to the floor and stay there for three to five seconds. If you have any back problems keep your knees slightly bent as you bend forward.

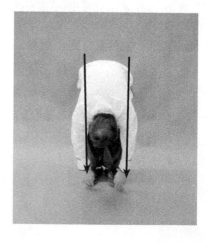

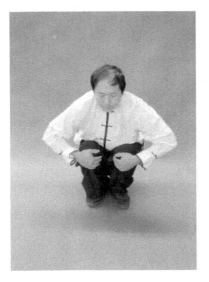

■ Finally, squat down with your feet flat on the floor to stretch your ankles. If you cannot keep your feet flat on the floor, use a lift under your heels.

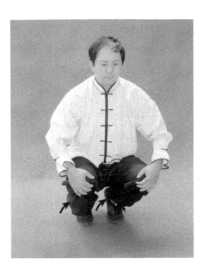

■ Next, lift your heels up to stretch the toes. Repeat the entire process ten times. After you finish, the inside of your body should feel very comfortable and warm.

Massaging the Large Intestine, Small Intestine, Urinary Bladder, and Kidneys

This exercise helps you to regain conscious control of the muscles in your abdomen. There are four major benefits to this abdominal exercise. First, when your lower dan tian (xia dan tian) area is loose, the qi can flow in and out easily. The lower dan tian is the main residence of your original qi (yuan qi). The qi in your dan tian can be led easily only when your abdomen is loose and relaxed. Second, when the abdominal area is loose, the qi circulation in the large and small intestines will be smooth, and they will be able to absorb nutrients and eliminate waste more efficiently. If your body does not eliminate effectively, the absorption of nutrients will be hindered, and you may become sick. Third, when the abdominal area is loose, the qi in the kidneys will circulate smoothly, and the original essence stored there can be converted more efficiently into qi. In addition, when the kidney area is loose, the kidney qi can be led downward and upward to nourish the entire body. Fourth, these exercises eliminate qi stagnation in the lower back, healing and preventing lower back pain.

- To practice this exercise, stand with your feet a comfortable distance apart and your knees slightly bent. As you get more used to this exercise and your legs become stronger, bend your knees a little bit more. Without moving your thighs or upper body, use the waist muscles to move the abdomen around in a horizontal circle. Circle in one 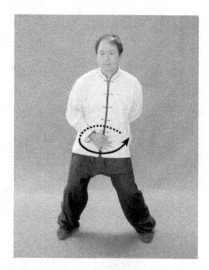 direction about ten times and then in the other direction about ten times. If you hold one hand over your lower dan tian and the other on your sacrum, you may be able to focus your attention better on the area you want to control.

In the beginning, you may have difficulty making your body move the way you want it to, but if you keep practicing, you will quickly learn how to do it. Once you can do the movement comfortably, make the circles larger and larger. Naturally, this will cause the muscles to tense somewhat and inhibit the qi flow, but the more you practice, the sooner you will be able to relax again. After you have practiced for a while and can control your waist muscles easily, start making the circles smaller and also start using your yi to lead the qi from the dan tian to move in these circles. The final goal is to have only a slight physical movement but a strong movement of qi.

When you practice, concentrate your mind on your abdomen, and inhale and exhale deeply and smoothly. Remember that breathing deep does not mean breathing heavily. When you breathe deep, keep the diaphragm and the muscles surrounding the lungs relaxed. Inhale to lead the qi into the center of the body and exhale to lead the qi out through the skin.

Massaging the Stomach, Liver, Spleen, Gallbladder, and Kidneys

Beneath your diaphragm is your stomach, to the right are your liver and gallbladder, to the left is your spleen, and in the back are your kidneys. Once you can comfortably do the circular movement in your lower abdomen, change the movement from horizontal to vertical and extend it up to your diaphragm. The easiest way to loosen the area around the diaphragm is to use a wavelike motion between the perineum and the diaphragm.

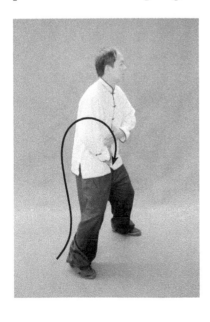

- You may find it helpful when you practice this to place one hand on your lower dan tian and your other hand above it with the thumb on the solar plexus. Use a forward and backward wavelike motion, flowing up to the diaphragm and down to the perineum and back. While you do this, inhale deeply when the motion is starting at the perineum and exhale as it reaches the diaphragm. Practice ten times.

- Next, continue the movement while turning your body slowly to one side and then to the other. This will slightly tense the muscles on one side and loosen them on the other, which will massage the internal organs. Repeat ten times.

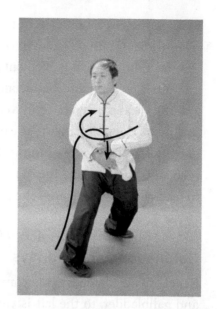

This exercise loosens the muscles around the stomach, liver, gallbladder, spleen, and kidneys and therefore improves the qi circulation there. It also trains you in using your mind to lead qi from your lower dan tian upward to the solar plexus area.

Massaging the Lungs and Heart

This exercise loosens up the chest and helps to regulate and improve the qi circulation in the lungs. According to the theory of the five elements in Chinese medicine, the lungs belong to the element known as metal (jin) while the heart belongs to the element fire (huo). Metal is able to cool down fire, and the lungs are able to regulate the qi of the heart. The heart is the most vital organ, and its condition is closely related to our life and death. If there is too much qi in the heart (when it is too yang), you speed up its degeneration and become prone to heart attacks. For this reason, qigong places great emphasis on using the lungs to regulate the qi in the heart. If we know how to relax the lungs and keep the qi circulating in them smoothly, they will be able to regulate the heart more efficiently.

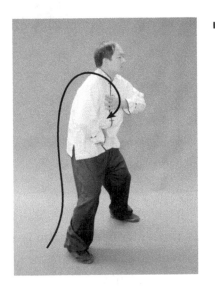

■ After loosening up the center portion of your body, extend the movement up to your chest. The wavelike movement starts in the abdomen, moves through the stomach, and up to the chest. You may find it easier to feel the movement if you hold one hand on your abdomen and the other lightly touching your chest. Do this movement ten times.

■ Next, extend the movement to your shoulders. Inhale when you move your shoulders backward and exhale when you move them forward. The inhalation and exhalation should be as deep as comfortably possible, and the entire chest should be very loose. Repeat the motion ten times.

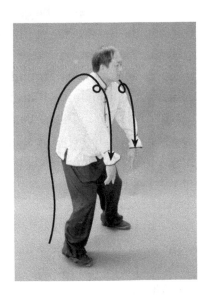

Massaging the Internal Organs with Your Hands

Using the hands to massage the internal organs is a natural human instinct, and we do it whenever we feel pain or qi stagnation in or near an organ. For example, if you have diarrhea and feel pain in your abdomen, you naturally massage yourself with your hand. Or if you overeat, you automatically stroke or rub your stomach with your palms to ease the pain.

- Laogong Cavity (P-8)

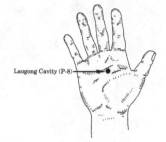

Laogong Cavity (P-8)

According to Chinese medicine, in the center of each palm is a cavity or gate called the laogong (P-8) that is used to regulate the qi of the heart whenever the qi flow is too strong. Unless you are sick, the qi in the heart is normally more positive than is necessary, especially in the summertime. When you are excited or nervous, even more qi accumulates around the heart. When this happens, the centers of your palms will feel warm and will often sweat.

Because the qi in the center of the palm is always strong, you can use this qi to help the stagnant organ qi to flow smoothly. Chinese physicians and qigong practitioners have developed a number of ways of using the hands to improve the qi circulation in the internal organs. In this section, we will introduce a few common ones that can be practiced easily by anyone. It is not true that only an expert can heal people with his or her hands. Anyone can do it with the proper knowledge.

Although it is best if you have someone else to massage you, because it is then easier for you to relax, many techniques can be self-applied effectively.

Abdomen

To massage your abdomen and regulate the qi circulation in your large and small intestines, place one hand on top of the other on your lower abdomen. If you are right-handed, it is better if you place your right hand on the bottom and the left hand on the top. Naturally, if you are left-handed, place the left hand on the bottom. The reason for this is quite simple: the qi is strongest in the hand you use most often, and it is easier for you to lead the qi from it.

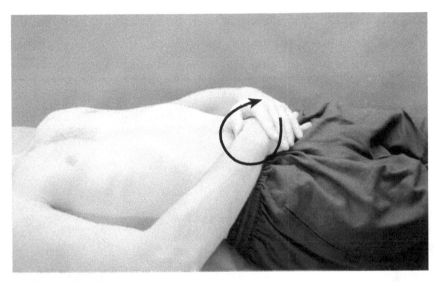

- When you massage your abdomen, it is best if you lie down so that your lower body is relaxed and the qi can circulate more easily and smoothly. Hold your hand lightly against the skin and place your other hand on top of it. Gently circle your hands clockwise, which is the direction of movement within the large intestine. Circling in the other direction would hinder the natural movements of peristalsis. Massage until you feel warm and comfortable deep inside your body.

As you massage, your breathing should be relaxed, deep, and comfortable. Place your mind a few inches under your palms. The mind will then be able to lead the qi inward to smooth out qi and blood stagnation.

Liver, Stomach, Spleen, and Gallbladder

In qigong massage for the internal organs, the liver, stomach, spleen, and gallbladder are usually included in the same techniques because they are all located in the middle of the front of the body. Maintaining healthy qi circulation in an organ requires not only that the circulation in the organ itself be smooth but also that the circulation between the organs be smooth. Therefore, when you massage these four internal organs, you should treat them as one instead of four.

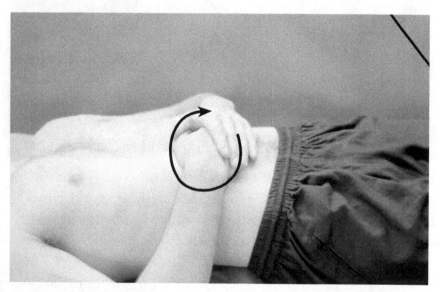

- Hold your hands as you did when massaging the lower abdomen, only now place them above the navel. Experience has shown that moving clockwise is again more effective than moving counterclockwise. It is easiest to do this massage when you are lying down. Massage until you feel warm inside.

Kidneys

Chinese medicine considers the kidneys to be perhaps the most important internal organs. The kidneys affect how the other organs function, so almost all forms of qigong place heavy emphasis on keeping them healthy.

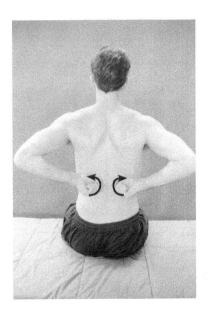

- To massage your own kidneys, close your hands into fists and place the thumb/index finger sides on your kidneys. Gently circle both fists until the kidneys are warm. In the summer, when your kidneys are normally too yang, it is desirable to dissipate some of the qi. This can be done by circling your right hand clockwise and your left hand counterclockwise. This leads the qi to the sides of your body. However, when you massage your kidneys in the wintertime, when the kidney qi is normally deficient (too yin), then you should reverse the direction and lead the qi to the center of your back to nourish the kidneys. As usual, the breathing and the mind are important keys to successful practice.

There are other methods of improving the qi circulation in the kidneys. One of the most common ones is to massage the bottoms of your feet. There is a qi gate in the front center of each sole that is called yongquan (K-1) (bubbling well). Massaging these two cavities will stimulate the qi circulation in the kidneys and help to regulate them.

- Yongquan Cavity

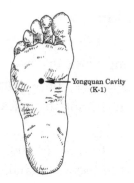

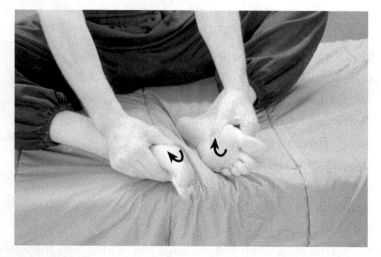

- Place your thumbs on your yongquan cavities and gently circle.

Lungs

As mentioned earlier, in the theory of the five elements, the lungs belong to metal (jin) while the heart belongs to fire (huo). According to this theory, the metal lungs can be used to regulate the heart fire just as metal can absorb heat. If you pay attention carefully, you will notice that when you feel heat around your heart due to excitement or even depression, you will normally thrust out your chest and greatly expand your lungs while inhaling. Doing this a few times reduces the pressure and the feeling of heat in the heart.

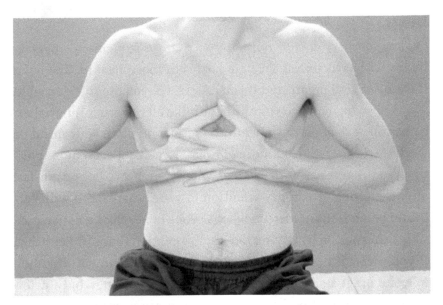

- To do qigong massage for your lungs, place both hands on the center of your chest just above the solar plexus. Inhale deeply.

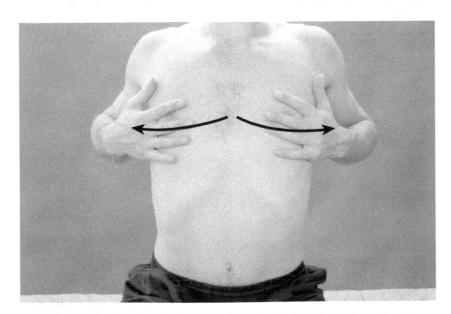

- Next, exhale while lightly pushing both hands to the sides. Do this until your lungs feel relaxed and comfortable. This massage is also good for the heart.

Heart

Qigong teachers do not normally encourage students to massage their own hearts unless they are fairly advanced in skill. The heart is the most vital organ, and if you mistreat it, you are in big trouble.

When you massage your heart, unlike all the other internal organs, you cannot place your mind on it. If you place your mind on your heart, you will lead more qi to it and make it even more positive. You may have noticed that when your heart is beating fast after exercising, if you pay attention to your heartbeat, it will start beating even faster. A person who is prone to heart attacks can possibly bring one on by paying too much attention to his or her heart. If your heart is beating too hard, the best thing is to pay attention to your lungs and breathe deeply and gently. After only a few breaths, your heart will slow down and regain its regular pace.

When you massage your heart, your mind should not be on your heart. Instead, keep your mind on the movement of your hands.

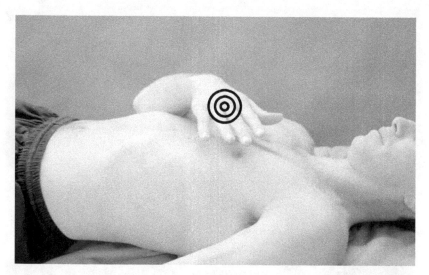

- To massage your heart, place your right hand over your heart at least three inches away from your chest. Move your hand in a small clockwise circle, and gradually increase the size of the circle. This takes the qi in the heart and spreads it out around the chest.

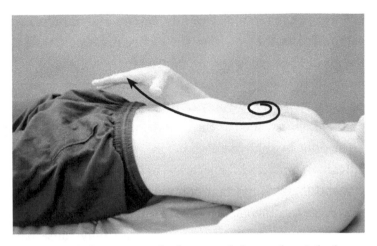

- Finally, lead the qi past the liver and down the right leg.

Testicles or Ovaries

Massaging the testicles or ovaries increases the production of hormones. According to Chinese muscle/tendon changing and marrow/brain washing qigong (yi jin jing and xi sui jing), massaging the testicles or ovaries correctly will increase hormone production and also increase the amount of qi led upward to the brain. Other effects are increasing the amount of qi stored in the body and strengthening the immune system. There are many ways to massage the testicles or ovaries. For example, if you massage your testicles, you may hold the testicles gently between your palms and circle your hands. You may also simply hold them in your hand and gently press and rub them. To massage ovaries, you may use the base knuckles of your pinkies to circle the ovaries gently. This subject is discussed in more detail in my book *Qigong—The Secret of Youth*.

3-3. Massage and Cavity Press (Acupressure)

Massage and cavity press (dian xue) are often used at the same time in treating arthritis. Massage is generally used first to loosen up the muscles and tendons around the joint and to increase the qi circulation. It lets the power of the cavity press penetrate deeper into the joint. Massage is also often used for acute pain.

In this section, we will introduce some of the more common and easy-to-learn techniques. Many of them you can do to yourself, although the majority, such as those done on the neck and the spine, need to be done by someone else. Before we discuss how to massage the individual joints and the location of the cavities, we would first like to mention one important point: when you are giving massage or cavity press treatments, you should not overstimulate the area or cavity (pressure point). Overstimulation can only cause pain and generate further stagnation of the qi and blood. In addition, too much pressure can further injure a joint that may be starting to heal. The purpose of massage and cavity press is to increase the qi and blood circulation, and anything that causes pain is incorrect.

Massage and Cavity Press Techniques

The first basic technique for massaging joints is to place a hand on the joint and rub gently back and forth or in circles until the area is warm.

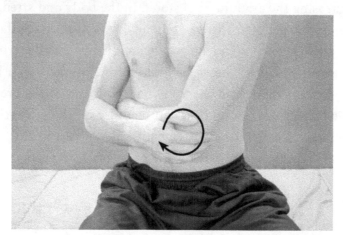

- Place your hand on the joint and rub gently back and forth or in circles until the area is warm. As the joint gets looser, you may increase the pressure as you rub so that the power penetrates deeper into the joint.

The second technique uses the middle joints of the fingers to massage.

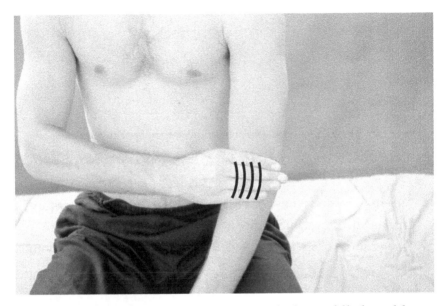

- Hold the area you are massaging with the middle knuckles of your fingers and be sure not to press the thumbs in and cause bruises. You want to feel the muscles and tendons, so apply gentle pressure and penetrate inward with your mind. Do not rub the skin. Instead, move your fingers back and forth and in circles to massage the muscles and tendons beneath the skin.

The third technique uses the thumb to rub or press and circle along the muscles and tendons of the joints.

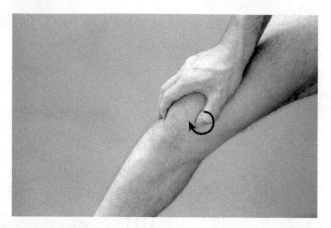

- Place your thumb on the joint and rub or press and circle along the muscles and tendons of the joint. The other four fingers are usually used to stabilize the thumb. This technique is used to increase the qi circulation and to lead the qi away from the joints.

The last basic technique uses the base of the palm.

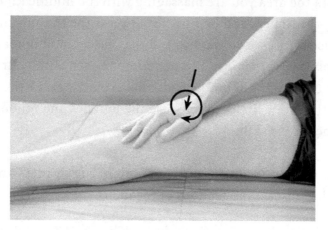

- Press your palm lightly inward to touch the muscles and tendons that you want to massage and then move your palm in circles. Do not rub the skin. After you have loosened one area, follow the muscle and tendon away from the joint and repeat the procedure. Adjust the pressure to control the depth of the massage and stimulate the various levels of muscle and tendon.

In cavity press, you use a fingertip to press directly on the cavity while concentrating deeply. The thumb, index, and middle fingers are most often used. Frequently, pressure is applied with a circular motion. If you are using your right hand, a clockwise motion usually nourishes the cavity while a counterclockwise one lowers the qi level. This is because a clockwise motion leads your yi (mind) forward and a counterclockwise motion leads your yi back. Naturally, if you are using your left hand, you circle counterclockwise to lead the qi forward and clockwise to lead it backward. Remember, your yi is the key to leading the qi forward and backward through your fingers.

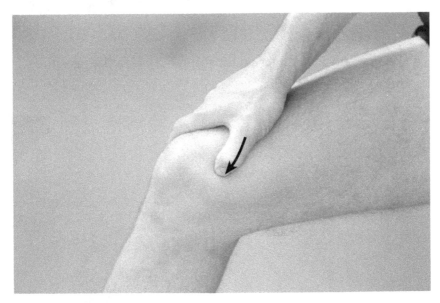

■ Press your thumb on the joint. Use the other fingers for support. Maintain the pressure for a few seconds.

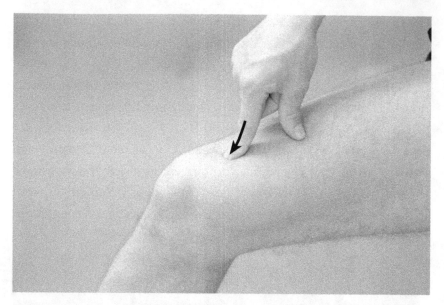

- Press your index finger on the joint. Maintain the pressure for a few seconds.

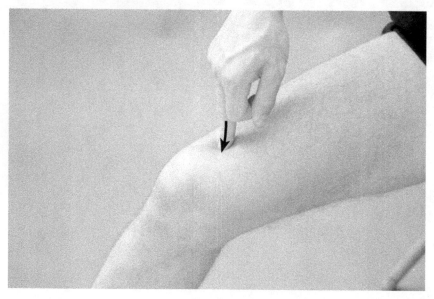

- You can also use your middle finger to press on the joint.

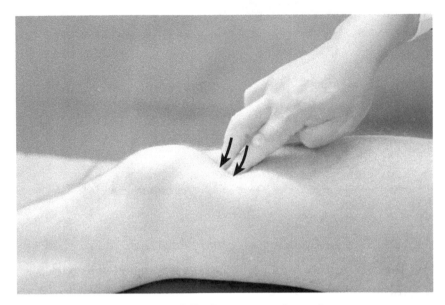

- Use the index and middle fingers together when more pressure is desired.

Basic Massage (Self and Partner)

In general, it is better to have someone massage you. When you massage yourself, it is difficult to be completely relaxed and concentrate on your breathing and the area being massaged. Also, it is impossible to do some neck and back massages on yourself.

The Neck and Spine

NECK

Massage (An Mo)
The main purpose of massaging the neck is to loosen the two main muscles in the back of the neck and to increase the qi circulation.

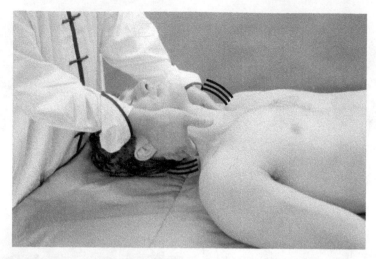

■ The best posture for a neck massage is lying on your back with the massager above your head.

An alternate way to receive a neck massage is to sit with the head pushed slightly back to relax the muscles. You may do this massage to yourself.

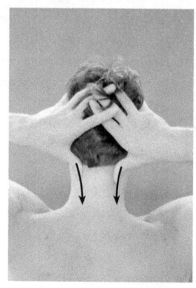

■ Starting at the top of the neck, rub downward with your thumbs.

Of course, it is easier and more comfortable if someone massages you.

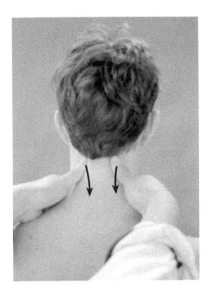

- Rub downward with the thumbs.

- Next, use the middle joints of your fingers to gently squeeze the muscles and move them around.

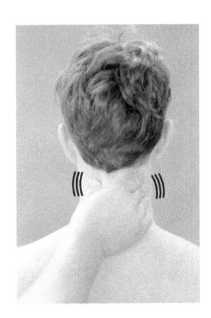

Cavity Press (Dian Xue)

There are six cavities that can be used to stimulate the qi circulation deep in the neck: fengfu (Gv-16), yamen (Gv-15), the two fengchi (GB-20) cavities, and the two tianzhu (B-10) cavities. The thumb and index finger are most commonly used. When doing this on yourself, first concentrate your mind and then gently press with a finger while keeping your neck relaxed. Press for three to five seconds and then let go. Five to ten presses are usually needed for proper stimulation. After doing the cavity press, place your attention deep inside the vertebrae and move your head around a few times.

■ Cavities on the Neck

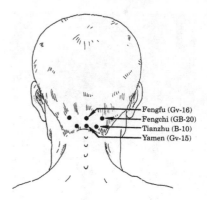

Fengfu (Gv-16)
Fengchi (GB-20)
Tianzhu (B-10)
Yamen (Gv-15)

SPINE

Massage (An Mo)

Obviously, you need to have someone else massage your back. Before you can loosen up the spine, you must first loosen up the trunk muscles. Therefore, start at the neck and gradually work downward. Do not massage upward, because this will lead the qi in the wrong direction and cause stagnation.

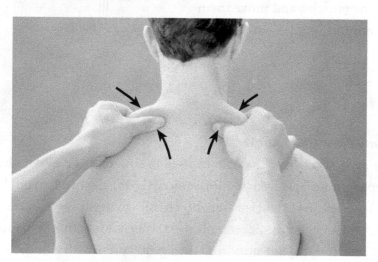

■ Loosen the neck muscles as explained above, then grab and gently squeeze the muscles between the neck and the shoulders. This will help lead the qi from the neck downward and spread it out across your back.

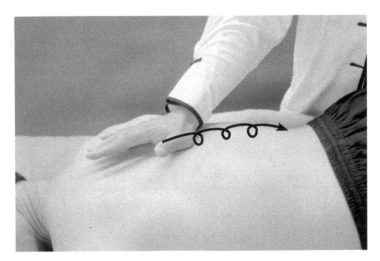

■ Next, use the base of your palm and massage downward in a circular motion. Massage from the neck down to the waist five to ten times.

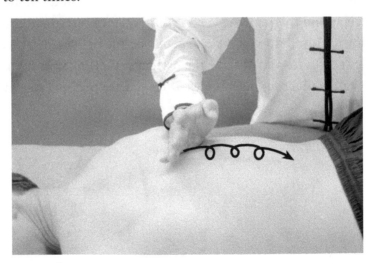

■ You could also use the edge of your palm to press the trunk muscles, moving downward with a circular massaging motion. Massage from the neck down to the waist five to ten times.

Once you have finished the circular pressing massage, place one hand on top of the other and press gently down on each joint in the spine. IMPORTANT: Do not press on the neck, and be sure that you press on the joints, not on the vertebrae. The purpose is to bend and loosen the joints a little. Press in coordination with the patient's breathing.

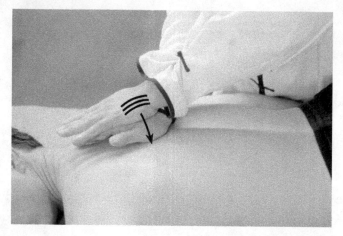

- Place your hands in position and ask your patient to inhale deeply and then exhale. When your patient is exhaling, press down. How hard you press depends on the patient. Start with light pressure and observe the patient's reaction. If he holds his breath and tenses his muscles, then you are pressing too hard.

Cavity Press (Dian Xue)

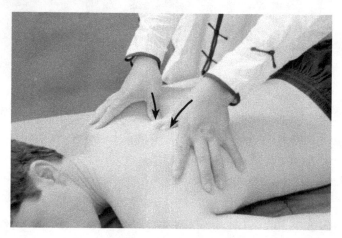

- Starting on the neck, press your thumbs into the gaps between the joints of the spine.

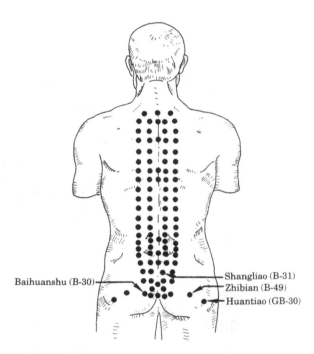

Baihuanshu (B-30)

Shangliao (B-31)
Zhibian (B-49)
Huantiao (GB-30)

■ Cavities on the Spine

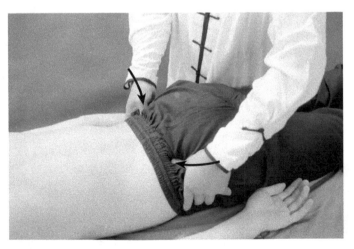

■ When you have reached the tailbone, press the shangliao
   (B-31), baihuanshu (B-30), zhibian (B-49), and huantiao
   (GB-30) cavities to lead the qi to the hips.

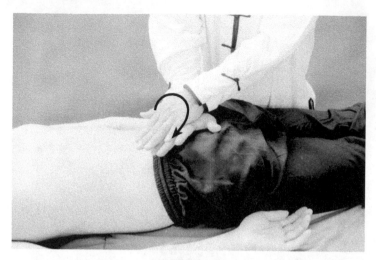

- Finally, use the base of the palm to gently massage the sacrum for three minutes.

After you have finished pressing on the sides of the spine, repeat the procedure, only now press about two inches away from the spine. Refer to the chart above on the cavities on the spine. It shows the cavities that should be pressed.

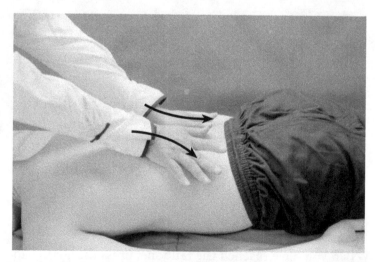

- After pressing, again use the palm to rub the trunk muscles, pushing to the sides and also downward. This procedure leads stagnant qi sideways and downward away from the spine.

WAIST

Massage (An Mo)

After you have massaged and loosened up the back, start on the kidneys. Good qi circulation in the kidneys is very important. When it is abnormal, the surrounding area will also be affected. It is best to have someone else massage your kidneys.

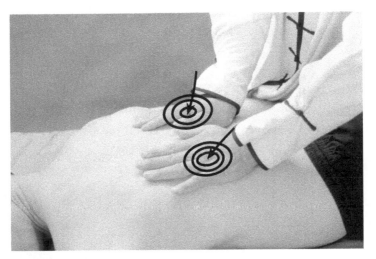

- To massage the kidneys, use the same circular motion discussed earlier. If you are massaging someone, you may also press gently down on the kidneys with your palms and then release the pressure. Do this about ten times, and you will feel the release of tension in the kidneys and an improvement in the qi circulation. Finally, use both palms to push from the kidneys to the sides of the body and also downward to the hips.

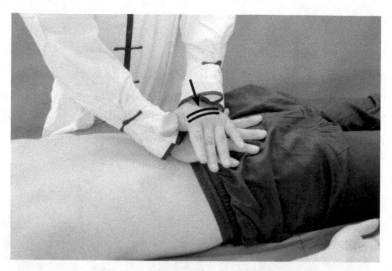

■ Next, press and release with your palms on the joint between the sacrum and the first vertebra about ten times.

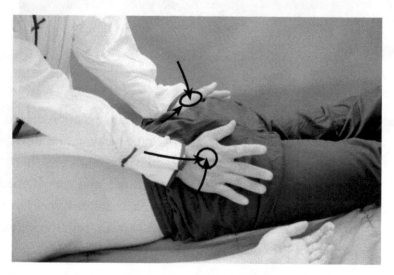

■ Next, push toward the sides and to the hips to lead the qi there.

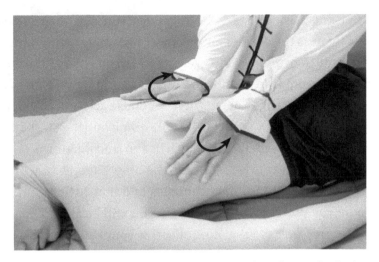

■ An alternative method is to place your hands on the kidneys or waist and move your hands in circles. Keep your hands in contact with the skin so that they lightly brush it, but don't let them rub the skin. Use very little pressure, so that the patient is comfortable and doesn't feel any pain.

Cavity Press (Dian Xue)

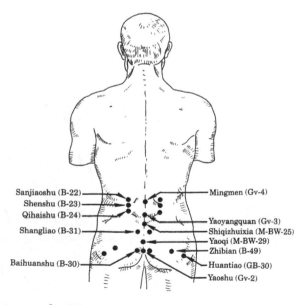

Sanjiaoshu (B-22)
Shenshu (B-23)
Qihaishu (B-24)
Shangliao (B-31)
Baihuanshu (B-30)

Mingmen (Gv-4)
Yaoyangquan (Gv-3)
Shiqizhuixia (M-BW-25)
Yaoqi (M-BW-29)
Zhibian (B-49)
Huantiao (GB-30)
Yaoshu (Gv-2)

■ Cavities on the Waist

After you have finished the massage, you can then use your thumbs to press the cavities on the lower back. Start with mingmen (Gv-4), and move down to yaoyangquan (Gv-3), shiqizhuixia (M-BW-25), yaoqi (M-BW-29), and finally yaoshu (Gv-2). Press each cavity three to five times, about three seconds each time. Next, press the sanjiaoshu (B-22), shenshu (B-23), qihaishu (B-24), shangliao (B-31), baihuanshu (B-30), zhibian (B-49), and huantiao (GB-30) cavities the same way to lead the qi to the hips. Experience will teach you the appropriate pressing techniques and how to apply pressure. The more you practice, the more easily you will be able to penetrate with your pressure, and the more effective your cavity press will be.

JOINTS IN THE LIMBS

In this section, we will discuss a few of the techniques used for massaging the joints in the limbs. Once you are familiar with them, you may use the same theory to create others. Remember that the goal of massage is to loosen up the muscles and tendons and to increase the qi circulation.

Massage (An Mo)

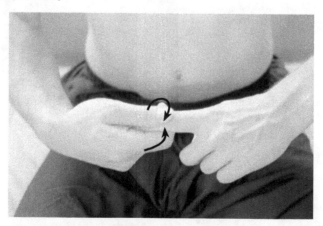

- Small joints such as in the fingers and toes can be held between the thumb and index finger while you apply circular pressure with the thumb. Move from one point to another until you have massaged the entire joint.

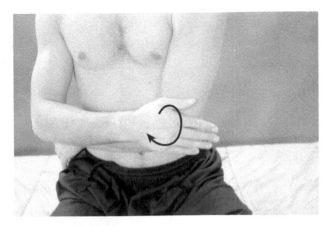

- With the bigger joints—wrists, knees, elbows, and shoulders—place your palm over the joint and massage in a circular motion until the joint is warm.

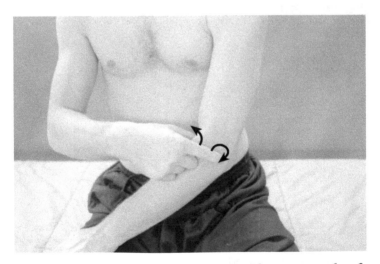

- You can then press and circle in particular areas with a finger or thumb to stimulate the qi circulation.

It is usually easier to have someone else massage your shoulder or hip.

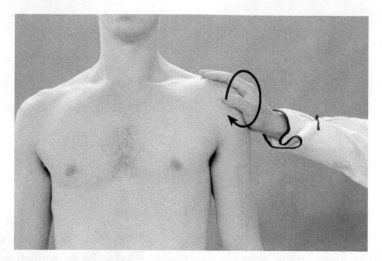

■ You can use the palm to massage the joints.

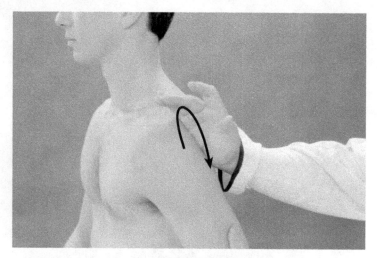

■ You can also use the edge of the palm.

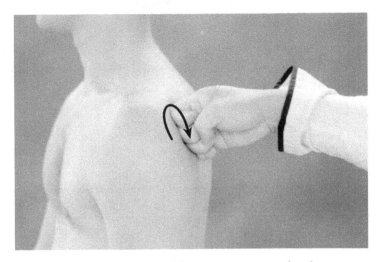

■ You can also use the knuckles to press in and rub.

These are only a few of the many techniques that can be used to massage the joints and increase the qi circulation. As you practice, you may discover many other ways to let your pressure penetrate deep into the joints.

Next, we will discuss the cavities or pressure points that are commonly used for cavity press. Some of them are not actually acupuncture cavities but rather places where finger pressure can easily penetrate deep into the joints.

Cavity Press (Dian Xue)

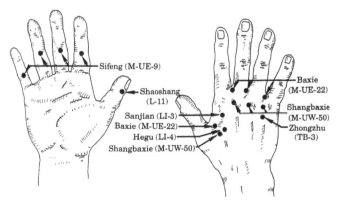

■ Cavities on the Hand

Hands (Fingers and Palms)

Hegu (LI-4), sanjian (LI-3), baxie (M-UE-22), sifeng (M-UE-9), shangbaxie (M-UE-50), shaoshang (L-11), shaoze (SI-1), laogong (P-8), and zhongzhu (TB-3).

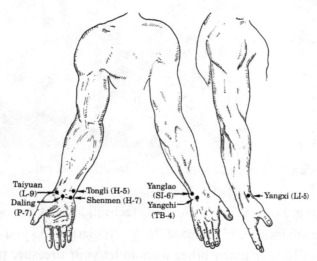

- Cavities on the Wrist

Wrists

Yangchi (TB-4), yanglao (SI-6), yangxi (LI-5), taiyuan (L-9), daling (P-7), shenmen (H-7), and tongli (H-5).

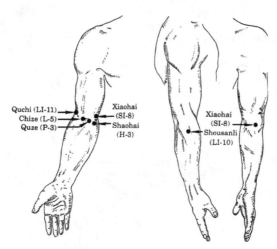

- Cavities on the Elbow

Elbows

Quchi (LI-11), shousanli (LI-10), chize (L-5), quze (P-3), shaohai (H-3), and xiaohai (SI-8).

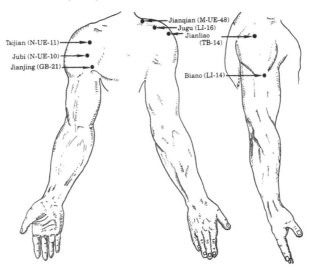

■ Cavities on the Shoulder

Shoulders

Jianqian (M-UE-48), jugu (LI-16), jianliao (TB-14), jubi (N-UE-10), taijian (N-UE-11), binao (LI-14), and jianjing (GB-21).

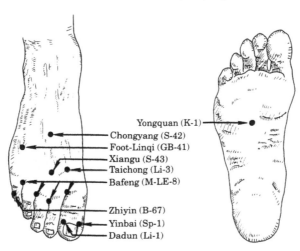

■ Cavities on the Foot

Toes and Feet

Chongyang (S-42), foot-linqi (GB-41), taichong (Li-3), xiangu (S-43), zhiyin (B-67), bafeng (M-LE-8), dadun (Li-1), yinbai (Sp-l), and yongquan (K-l).

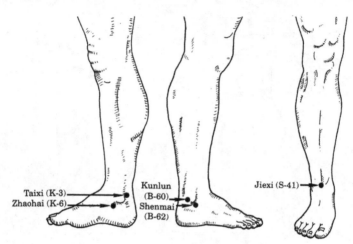

■ Cavities on the Ankle

Ankles

Jiexi (S-41), zhaohai (K-6), taixi (K-3), kunlun (B-60), and shenmai (B-62).

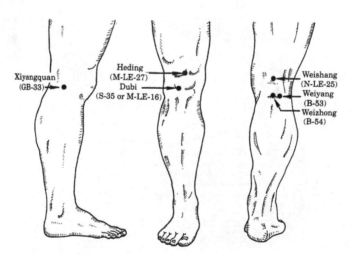

■ Cavities on the Knee

Knees

Dubi (S-35 or M-LE-16), heding (M-LE-27), xiyangquan (GB-33), weizhong (B-54), weiyang (B-53), and weishang (N-LE-25).

Femur-Juliao (GB-29)

Huantiao (GB-30)

■ Cavities on the Hip

Hips

Femur-juliao (GB-29) and huantiao (GB-30).

3-4. Qigong Exercises for Arthritis

Before introducing the qigong exercises, we would first like to discuss the best time to practice qigong. Experience indicates that the best time is in the early morning. The pain and stiffness of arthritis are most severe in the early morning because the qi is most stagnant. If you can do some massage and some qigong, you should be able to remove the stagnation and lessen the discomfort for the rest of the day. Therefore, in the early morning you should gently and lightly massage the joints until they are warm and the qi circulation has increased, and then gradually and gently start the qigong exercises.

You should also do the exercises right before you go to bed to smooth out any qi stagnation. This will speed up the repair and healing of the joints while you sleep and also lessen pain and stiffness the next morning. If you are able, you may add another practice session in the afternoon. Normally, your qi is the strongest in the afternoon. You may take advantage of this to do qigong exercises and lead qi to the joints. Naturally, if you have the time, you may do the qigong exercises whenever you can.

There are a few things you should be aware of. First, when the joint is inflamed, you should not get involved in heavy qigong exercise. Gently massage the joint to increase the qi circulation, and then do some light and easy exercises. Second, when you have the least pain and stiffness, take advantage of the opportunity and practice a little more than usual. Third, do not overdo it. The way to judge this is that if about two hours after practice you still feel significant pain, then it was probably too much. The next time, you should reduce the number of repetitions. With a little experience, you will soon be able to judge what is right for you. Practice a comfortable length of time and gradually increase the number of repetitions. Fourth, you should minimize the stress directly on the affected joints. As mentioned earlier, the best and most effective way is to bring the practice into your daily life and let it become a habit.

In this section, we will introduce a number of qigong exercises that can be used to heal arthritis and rebuild the joints. Remember that the key to healing and regrowth is leading qi to the joints and helping it to circulate smoothly there. The main way to do this is to concentrate your attention totally on the area you are exercising. When you concentrate, your yi (mind) leads qi to the joint. Breathing calmly and deeply also helps you to lead the qi inward into the organs, joints, and bone marrow. Once you have grasped these tricks, you will be able to use the qigong movements to circulate qi in the joint smoothly and strongly.

When you practice, you should wear warm clothing and avoid exposing your joints to cold air or wind. After you practice, you should cover the joints and keep them warm. Remember that everyone is different, and you have to use your common sense to judge what is best for you.

When you are just starting these qigong exercises, remember that you should not focus on building up the muscles and tendons. If you do this, your concentration will cause them to tense. This will increase the pressure in the joint and may cause the bones to grind against each other, which will hinder the healing process. Furthermore, although exercising the muscles and tendons may lead qi to the joints, if you exercise too strenuously you will cause tension, which will stagnate the qi circulation. You should always remember that the key to good qigong is using the mind and gentle movements to lead qi to the joints and increase smooth qi circulation.

Once you have repaired some of the joint damage, you can then gradually start to emphasize strengthening the muscles and tendons. When the joints, muscles, and tendons are healthy, you have cured the arthritis. Remember that the strength of the joints must be built slowly and gradually. Do not expect to rebuild them in one night, one week, or even one month. However, after three months of consistent practice, you should start to see improvement.

CHAPTER 4

Qigong Exercises

4-1. The Trunk

Neck

The neck is the passageway to the brain for the qi and blood. The brain is the center of your whole being, so if the circulation of the qi and blood is stagnant or blocked, your brain will not receive the proper nourishment. This causes dizziness, headache, and, in the long term, memory loss and accelerated aging. Blockages of the circulation to the head are often caused by neck injuries or arthritis in the neck joints. You can see that in order to keep your brain functioning healthily, the first step is to remove any blockages of the circulation in the neck. The next two exercises are commonly used in China for this purpose.

Look Left and Right (Zuo Gu You Pan)

This exercise can be done with the eyes open or closed, as long as you are able to concentrate your mind on your neck. Keep your mind calm, concentrate on what you are doing, and feel the movement of the joints. The more you concentrate, the deeper you will lead the qi. The exercise is very simple.

- Turn your head slowly from one side to the other. You may sit or stand. As you turn your head to the side, exhale, and as you turn your head back to the front, inhale. Keep your neck as relaxed as possible. Keep turning your head until your neck starts getting warm, which may take twenty to fifty turns.

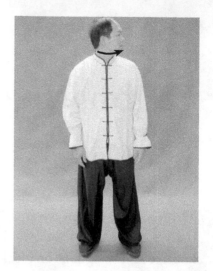

The Heaven Spins and the Earth Turns (Tian Xuan Di Zhuan)

After you have finished the head-turning exercise, continue by rotating your head. Remember, the circle should be small. Large circles may cause the neck vertebra to grind into each other, which will make the problem worse. Stay relaxed and concentrated.

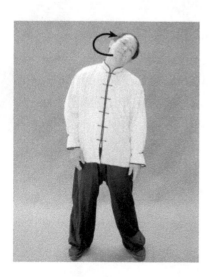

- Rotate your head clockwise about twenty to fifty times and then counterclockwise another twenty to fifty times. Rotate your head the same number of times in both directions. When you have finished, close your eyes, keep your mind calm, and feel the qi flowing in your neck area for a few minutes.

4-2. Spine

According to Chinese medicine, there is a qi vessel called the governing vessel (du mai), which follows the spine upward to the back of your head. Any problem with the spine can cause muscle tension, which, in turn, can cause stagnation of the qi flow in the governing vessel. The governing vessel controls the six yang primary qi channels in the body (large intestine, small intestine, triple burner, urinary bladder, gallbladder, and stomach channels). When there is any problem with the qi circulation in the governing vessel, the six yang primary channels and their related organs will also be affected.

Because any problem with your spine directly affects your health, Chinese qigong pays much attention to strengthening the spine and maintaining the qi circulation in the back. The following movements are only some of the exercises that can be used to strengthen and maintain qi circulation in the spine and back.

Large Dragon Softens Its Body (Da Long Ruan Shen)

This exercise is a wavelike movement that starts at the legs and flows upward to the sacrum and finishes at the neck.

- The movement goes from side to side or forward and backward—or you can do both. You may interlock your hands and move them along with your body. Keep your attention on your spine, where the movement is. You may also do this exercise sitting down, in which case, you generate the movement in your abdomen and let it flow upward. The body remains as relaxed as possible. Practice from twenty to fifty times until the spine feels warm.

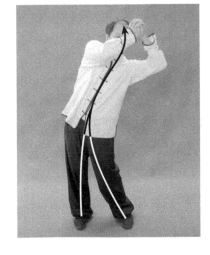

Large Dragon Turns Its Body (Da Long Zhuan Shen)

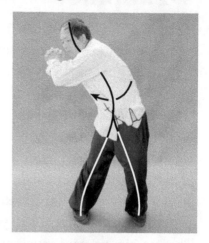

- Continue the wave movement described above, only now also start turning from side to side. The turning uses the trunk muscles to rotate the vertebrae, which increases the mobility of the spine.

Waist

Be very careful when you exercise your waist. Moving too vigorously can injure the lower back and spine, so proceed slowly and carefully. The following three qigong exercises can improve qi circulation around the waist.

Rotating the Waist (Niu Yao Xian Huo)

This is a very simple exercise.

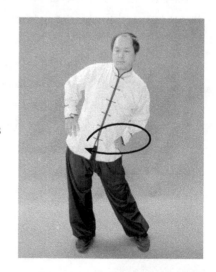

- Keep your head and feet in place as you gently and smoothly move your waist in a circle. Circle ten to twenty times in one direction, and then repeat the same in the other direction. As you practice, pay attention to the waist area and try to feel the movement inside your body. When you can feel the movement of your spine, it means that you are leading qi to it and at the same time using the motion to circulate the qi.

Lion Rotates Its Head (Shi Zi Yao Tou)

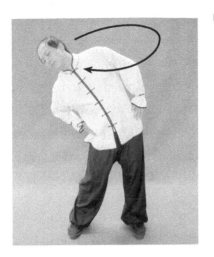

- In this exercise, keep your legs and waist in place and swing your upper body in a circle. Move in one direction ten to twenty times, and then move in the reverse direction the same number of times. Remember to move gently. Your mind is always the key to success. You may also do this exercise while sitting on a chair.

Bend and Straighten the Waist (Qian Gong Hou Ju)

This is one of the easiest qigong exercises. In Chinese wai dan qigong, it is commonly used to massage the kidneys by tensing and relaxing the back muscles. It is also used to clear up waist problems and lower back pain.

- To do this exercise, simply relax your body as much as possible and bend forward. Gently swing your hips from side to side. Stay bent over for about five seconds and then gently straighten up. Repeat ten to twenty times. Once your waist has regained its strength, you may increase the number of repetitions. As always, keep your mind on the area being exercised.

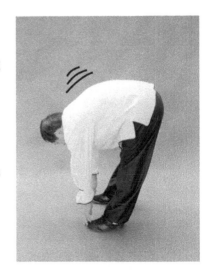

4-3. Limbs

Arms

Hands (Fingers and Palms)

Usually when you exercise your fingers, your palms are also involved. In addition, because they are all connected, whenever you exercise your hands, you are also to some degree exercising your wrists.

Chinese physicians have found that people who use their hands and fingers a lot are sick less often than people who don't. The reason for this is very simple. There are six primary qi channels that connect the fingers to six of your internal organs. Whenever you work with your hands, you build up qi in those channels, and this qi then flows into and nourishes the internal organs. There are many qigong exercises for the hands. We will present four of them.

Swimming Octopus (Zhang Yu You Shui)

This exercise also includes the wrists. If you wish, you may practice this one hand at a time.

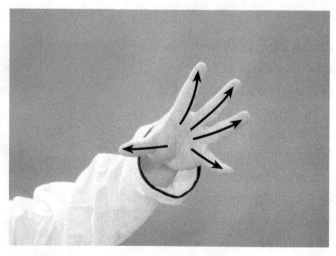

- Stretch your hands forward while spreading out the fingers. The wrist joint is also opened and stretched.

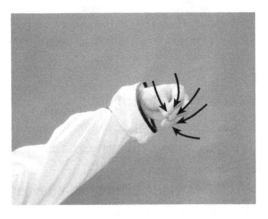

- Next, draw your wrists back while closing the fingers.

Move your hands in and out, opening and closing the hands so that they look like a swimming octopus. After doing this movement thirty to fifty times, your fingers, palms, and wrists will usually feel very warm. Remember, when you practice, your hands should remain as relaxed as possible, and your mind should be concentrated on them.

Flying Finger Waves Gong (Zhi Bo Xiang Gong)

This exercise is used by the Crane style of gongfu to strengthen the palms and the base of the fingers.

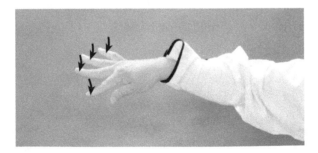

- Bend your thumbs and fingers one after the other and then straighten them one at a time, repeating the motion in a sort of wave. Only bend the knuckles closest to the hands. If you bend the other knuckles you will fail to develop the base of the fingers. After you have done twenty to fifty repetitions, your palms and the base of your fingers should feel very warm and perhaps a little sore.

After practicing, relax your arms as much as possible to allow the qi that has accumulated in your hands to circulate to your arms and body.

Tiger Claw Training (Hu Zhua Xing Gong)

This exercise originated with the Tiger Claw style of gongfu and is more strenuous than the previous ones. This means that you should be more careful about how much tension you generate during practice. If your arthritis is very serious, you should probably not tense your muscles until your condition has improved, and then you should increase the tension very gradually.

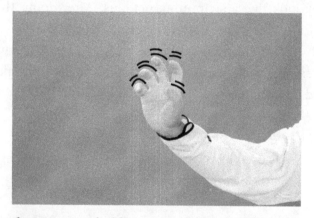

- To do this exercise, hold your hands like a tiger's paws.

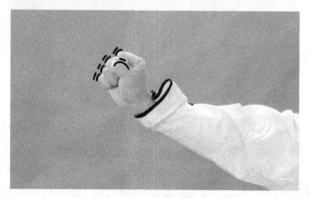

- Gradually pull all of your fingers in to the center of the palms, and then open your hands again to the tiger's paw shape. After twenty to fifty repetitions, your fingers and palms should be very warm.

When you are finished, relax your arms and allow the qi to flow freely upward into your body.

Rolling the Taiji Ball (Zhuan Taiji Qiu)

In China, taiji balls are well known for their role in curing many illnesses, such as irregular qi circulation in the six primary channels, and also local problems such as arthritis. Many arthritis patients have used taiji balls to cure arthritis in the fingers and palms and to strengthen their joints. Taiji ball training for arthritis in the hands is very simple.

Martial taiji practitioners do a variety of exercises with various sizes of balls. However, the balls used for treating arthritis in the hands and wrists usually have a diameter of about one and one-half inches. In ancient times, the balls were made of wood. Nowadays, however, they are made of metal, which is stronger and lasts longer. Metal taiji balls can be purchased in most Chinese department stores or martial art supplies stores.

- Hold two of the balls in one hand and move them in a circle with your fingers to rotate them. Your hands should feel warm after only five to ten minutes.

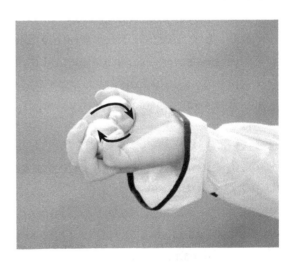

If you are patient and practice three or four times a day, you should see improvement in your arthritic condition in only a few months. Once your arthritis has improved, you may start rebuilding the strength of your muscles by increasing the tension in your hands as you do the following exercises.

Wrists

Rotating the Wrists (Zhuan Wan)

Rotating your wrists is very simple.

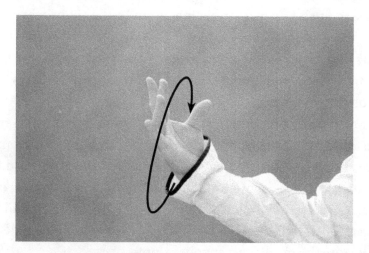

- Relax your wrists and move your hands in circles. Keep your attention on your wrists to feel the rotation and make it as smooth as possible. Keep rotating until your wrists are warm, and then reverse the rotation and do the same number of repetitions. It usually takes three hundred or more rotations before your wrists start to feel warm, especially in the wintertime.

Rotating the Wrists with Interlocked Fingers (Jiao Zhi Zhuan Wan)

This exercise is similar to the previous one, only now the hands are interlocked and help each other. Once you have rebuilt your joints, this exercise can also be very helpful in rebuilding the tendons and muscles in your wrists. To do this, simply increase the tension on the wrists.

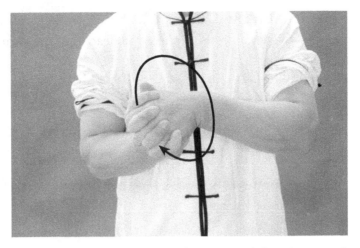

- Lace your fingers together and move both hands in circles. Keep your attention on your wrists, and practice the same number of times in either direction.

Rotating the Wrists while Holding Hands (Jiao Shou Zhuan Wan)

This exercise is very similar to the previous one.

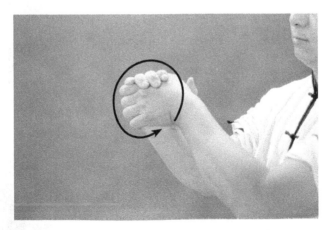

- In this exercise, instead of interlocking your fingers, your hands are grasping each other. Again, keep your mind on your wrists and feel what is going on there. Once you have rebuilt the joints, you can increase the pressure to strengthen the tendons and muscles.

As you can see, the exercises are quite simple. You can easily discover other movements or exercises that lead qi to the joints and increase their strength.

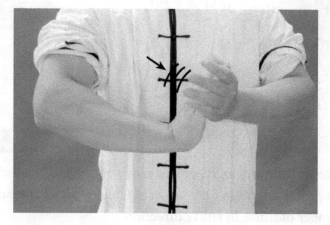

- For example, you can simply hold one hand steady and push it with the other one, and then relax. Push and relax until the wrist of the pushing hand starts to get warm.

Elbows

Lifting Movement (Shang Ti Wan Zhou)

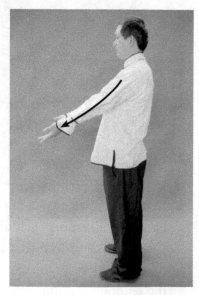

- Extend your arms out in front of you with the palms up as if you are holding something.

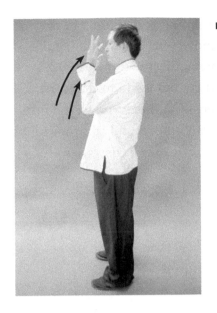

■ Raise your hands up to your face and then lower them. Keep your mind on your elbows and practice until they are warm. Then practice the same movement with the palms facing down. Once you are comfortable with this exercise, you can do it holding books or other light objects in your hands.

Sideward Movement (Nei Wai Wan Zhou)

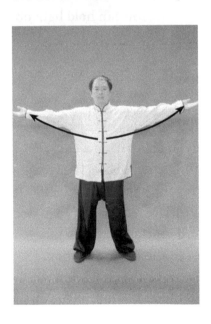

■ Extend your arms to the sides with the palms facing upward.

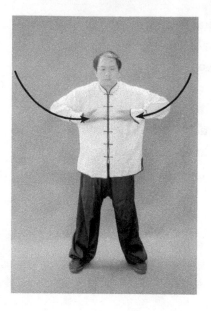

- Keeping your elbows in place, move your hands in to touch your chest and then swing them out again to the starting position. Keep your mind on your elbows and continue to practice until they are warm.

Then turn your palms down and repeat the same movement. Once you are comfortable with the exercise, you can hold light objects in your hands as you practice.

Rotating the Elbows (Zhuan Zhou)

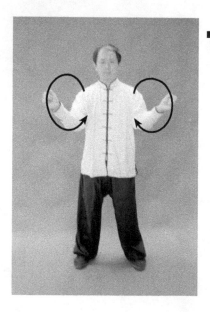

- Hold your arms in front of you as if you are driving a car. Keeping your elbows in place, move your hands in circles. Start with fifty repetitions of an inward motion and then fifty times in the other direction. Don't make the circles too big, as this will put too much tension on the tendons in the elbows.

Shoulders

Rotating the Shoulders (Song Jian)

- Use your shoulder muscles to move both shoulder joints around. First circle forward about fifty times and then reverse the circling motion for another fifty times. Keep your mind on your shoulders, and keep them as relaxed as possible. Don't move too fast or you will cause muscle tension, which can hinder the qi circulation.

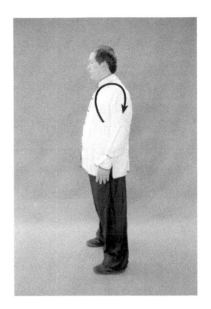

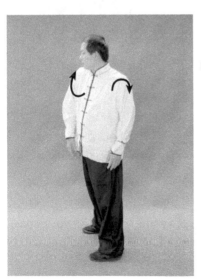

- You may also circle your shoulders with one of them 180 degrees behind the other. This motion has the advantage of moving your chest more, which increases the qi circulation in the shoulders and helps any stagnant qi there spread to the chest.

Front Waving (Qian Bo)

This exercise comes from Crane martial qigong. Move your arms like a crane's wings when it is flying. It is believed that cranes can fly long distances without rest because they know the key to circulating qi in the joints where the wings connect to the body. Crane gongfu emphasizes the shoulders in its qigong training. This waving exercise is only one of many, but it is a key one in developing the qi circulation and rebuilding the shoulder joints.

The key to success is relaxing your shoulder joints as much as possible and moving your arms and chest together. If you can do this, the muscles and tendons in the shoulders will be very relaxed and the qi circulation will be smooth.

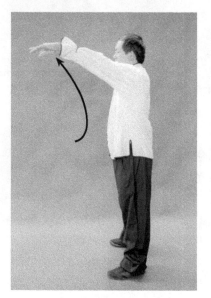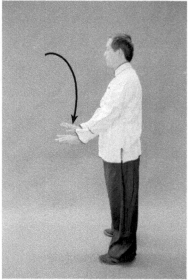

- To do front waving, simply extend both arms in front of your chest and wave them up and down like flying wings. You may move both arms up and down simultaneously.

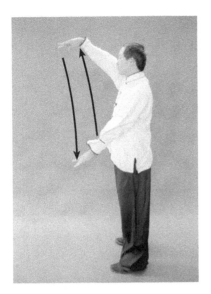

- You may also alternate your arms, moving one up and the other one down.

Crane Flying (He Xiang)

Crane flying also comes from Crane-style qigong. As in the previous form, treat your arms and chest as one unit and relax the shoulders to their maximum. You should fly until your arms are warm.

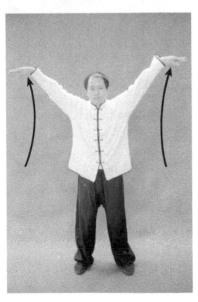
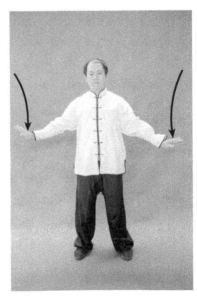

- Extend your wings (arms) to your sides as they are on the bird. You may move both arms up and down at the same time, or alternately move one up and the other one down.

If you train consistently, after a few months you will be able to increase the number of wing strokes to several hundred without feeling tired. This means that you will have rebuilt your shoulder joints. If you are interested in knowing more about soft White Crane qigong, please refer to my book *The Essence of Shaolin White Crane*.

Front-Back Swinging Arms (Qian Hou Shuai Bi)

This exercise is adopted from the way your hands naturally swing while you are walking.

- Simply drop your arms naturally and comfortably beside your body, then swing one arm forward while the other swings backward. Turn your body from side to side and let your arms swing naturally. Swing them somewhat higher than you do when walking.

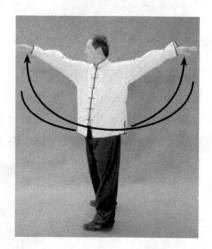

Alternatively, you may swing both arms forward and backward together.

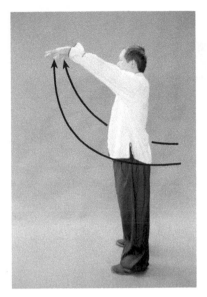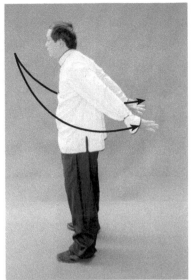

- Arm-swinging qigong has become very popular in Taiwan in the last twenty years because it has been proven to cure many kinds of illnesses, especially those related to the lungs and heart. Naturally, this exercise is also used for treating arthritis in the shoulders.

Front-Side Swing Arms (Qian Ce Shuai Bi)

This exercise is very similar to the previous one; however, it comes from martial Crane qigong. In this exercise, you swing your arms in an undulating motion to the front and to the sides.

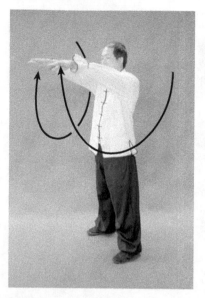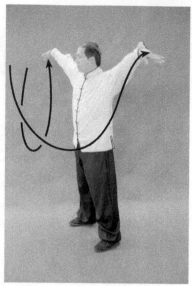

- You may swing both arms at the same time. Swing them forward and then sideward.

You may also alternate arms, swinging one forward and the other sideward. Extend your fingers but keep them relaxed. Keep your wrists relaxed too, so that they move slightly behind the arms.

After you have rebuilt your shoulder joints, you may start to strengthen your muscles and tendons. You can do this by holding a weight in your hands while you are doing the exercises. Start with a light weight and gradually increase it.

Legs

People in China know that walking is one of the most effective exercises for curing arthritis in the shoulders, hips, knees, and ankles. When you walk, your mind is peaceful and your body is relaxed. As you walk, pay attention to your stability, balance, and the motion of your joints. Swing your arms smoothly and lift your legs a little higher than usual. Start walking a mile or so, and increase the distance gradually as you get used to it. When the weather is too cold, or when it is raining, you can walk in place instead. When you feel comfortable walking, you can start walking uphill. On days when you can't go outside, you can walk up and down stairs. In China, when a patient has started walking again, physicians will frequently encourage him or her to walk up a hill in the morning, do some qigong exercises, and then walk home.

In addition to walking, there are several other qigong exercises that can be used to cure arthritis in the legs.

Toes

Squeeze the Toes (Ji Jiao Zhi)

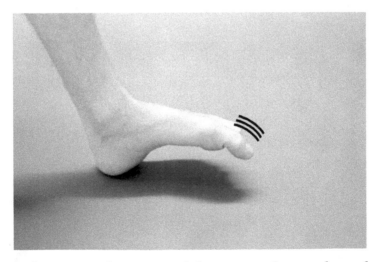

- Bend your toes down toward the centers of your soles and hold them there for about three seconds, and then relax. Keep your mind on the joints of the toes, and repeat the exercise until they are warm.

Up and Down Movements (Ding Zhi)

- Stand up on your toes for three to five seconds and then lower yourself down onto your feet. Keep your mind on the joints of your toes, and repeat the exercise until they are warm.

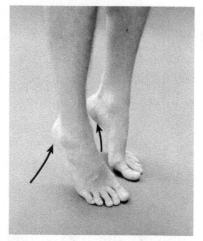

This exercise is also very beneficial for arthritis in the ankles.

Walking on the Toes (Zhi Xing)

This is the simplest exercise for the toes, feet, and ankles.

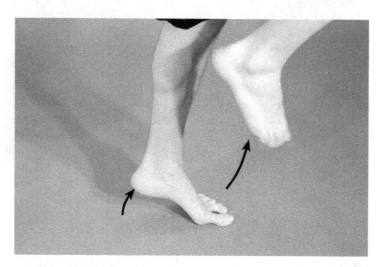

- Simply walk on your toes while paying attention to your feet. Walk slowly, keeping your body centered and balanced. After you walk about one hundred steps, your feet will feel warm. You may then sit down and allow the qi and blood to circulate upward. After you have rested for a while, you may repeat the exercise.

Ankles

In addition to some of the toe exercises that are also beneficial for the ankles, there is another common qigong exercise that can be used to improve the qi and blood circulation in your ankles.

Rotating the Ankles (Zhuan Hua Guan Jie)

If you are able, stand with your weight on one leg and move the ankle of the other leg in a circle. If you need to, you may use a wall or table for support.

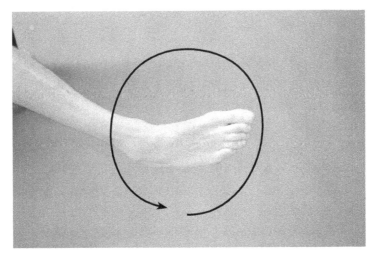

- Circle in one direction thirty times and then reverse the direction and circle another thirty times. If you cannot do this exercise standing, you may do it sitting. Exercise slowly and pay attention to the movement of the joints so that you can feel the qi moving there.

Knees

Straighten and Bend Movement (Wan Xi)

When you do this exercise, you may stand on one leg, or you may sit on the edge of a chair.

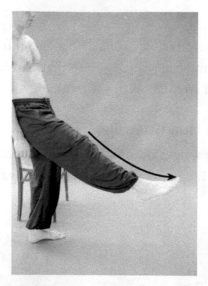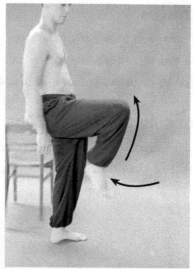

- Stand on one leg. Slowly straighten out the other leg in front of you and then bend it. Repeat the exercise until the knee is warm, and then do the same number of repetitions with the other leg.

Remember, it is your mind that leads the qi to the joint, so keep your mind on the exercising joint and feel deeply into it. This way, the qi will be led deep into the joint. Once your knees are healthy again, you can start strengthening the muscles and tendons by placing a weight on your ankles as you exercise.

Moving the Body Up and Down (Xia Dun Shang Li)

When you start doing this exercise, if your knees are weak and give you pain, bend them only a little. Only when the strength of your knees has been rebuilt should you start squatting lower.

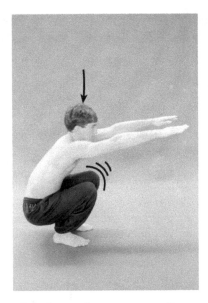 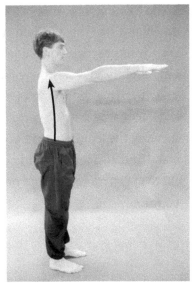

- Bend your knees, squat down, then stand up. Do the exercise slowly and keep your mind on your knees. Again, if your knees are weak, squat only a little.

Horse Stance Training (Ma Bu)

Horse stance training is widely used in the Chinese martial arts to strengthen the knees. Arthritis patients whose knees are not very strong should proceed very cautiously with this exercise. Horse stance training is one of the most effective techniques for rebuilding the muscles and tendons in the knees.

- To do horse stance, simply squat down and stay there. When you start your practice, squat down only slightly, and stay there for only twenty seconds or so. Once the knees are stronger, you can increase the length of time you stand and also lower your body more to put more pressure on your knees.

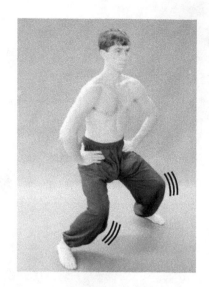

Hips

Raise and Lower the Leg (Shang Xia Ti Jiao)

If possible, stand on one leg. Use a wall or table for support if necessary.

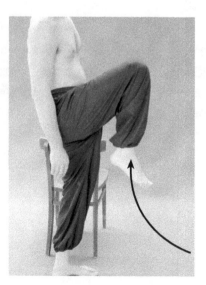 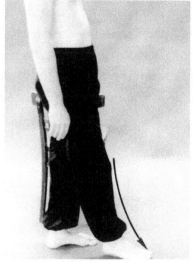

- Simply raise one leg and then lower it. Repeat thirty times and then change legs. Keep your mind on your hip joints and do the exercise slowly.

Sideward Motion and Rotating the Hip
(Zuo You Zhuan Tun)

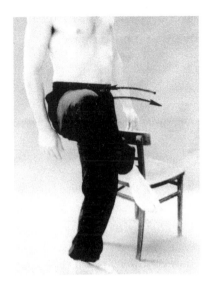

■ If you are able to stand on one leg and lift the other leg easily, move the knee of the lifted leg side to side ten times. Keep your mind on the hip joint.

■ Next, move the knee in a circle ten times in each direction. Move slowly at first. When the joints are strong again, you can increase the speed. Keep your mind on the hip joint.

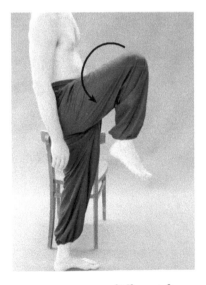

You can see that these qigong exercises are not very different from the exercises you are already familiar with. What makes them different is that you are not just making a physical motion; you are also using your mind and attention to lead qi to the joint to repair the damage and strengthen the muscles and tendons. You are also inhaling and exhaling deeply to move the qi more efficiently into the joints and increase the qi circulation. It is also important that you move slowly. This keeps the muscles and tendons relaxed and allows the qi to move more freely to the joint. When you move slowly, it is also easier for you to keep your mind on the joint and to feel deep inside it. Faster motions are harder to control and can easily cause more damage.

Conclusion

WHEN YOU PRACTICE Chinese qigong, understanding the theory and principles is as important as the exercises themselves. If you understand the theory and principles, your mind will not doubt. Only when you feel confident about what you are doing will you continue to practice. Furthermore, if you understand the theory and principles, you can create variations or newer exercises that may suit you better and yield better results. It is not uncommon for people who do not understand the theory and principles to practice qigong blindly and cause further injury. Therefore, when you practice qigong, you should study and ponder its theory and principles.

Another thing you should realize is no one can understand you, especially mentally, better than you can understand yourself. The best way to heal yourself is to know yourself and understand the key to your individual problem. Then you can adapt the recommended methods to fit your particular problem and your personality. If you can do this, then the qigong exercises that can benefit you will be naturally carried over into your lifestyle and become part of your life. This is the only way you will continue to practice and the only way the benefits will really last.

As I mentioned in the beginning of this book, Chinese medicine has many ways of treating arthritis, and I know only a few of them. I hope people who are qualified in other fields such as acupuncture and herbal treatment will contribute their knowledge and experience to fill this void.

In addition to introducing the West to the qigong exercises for healing arthritis, I have had another goal in writing this book. I sincerely hope this book will gain the attention of the Western medical establishment and encourage them to become involved in qigong experimentation, study, and research. This book is not an authority on this subject. It is, however, an attempt to open communication between East and West on the subject of medicine and healing. I deeply believe that if all of the different cultures can share their knowledge and experience and cooperate with one another, medical science will take a great step forward for the benefit of all humankind.

Translation and Glossary of Chinese Terms

an mo. Literally, press rub. Together they mean massage.

Ba Duan Jin. Eight Pieces of Brocade. A wai dan qigong practice that is said to have been created by Marshal Yue Fei during the Southern Song dynasty (1127–1279 CE).

ba mai. Referred to as the eight extraordinary vessels. These eight vessels are considered to be qi reservoirs that regulate the qi status in the primary qi channels.

bafeng (M-LE-8). Eight winds. The name of eight acupuncture cavities that belong to the "miscellaneous points."

baihuanshu (B-30). White circle's hollow. The name of an acupuncture point that belongs to the bladder channel.

baxie (M-UE-22). Eight evils. The name of eight acupuncture cavities that belong to the miscellaneous points.

binao (LI-14). Arm and scapula. The name of an acupuncture cavity that belongs to the large intestine channel.

changqiang (Gv-1). Long strength. The name of an acupuncture cavity that belongs to the governing vessel.

Cheng, Gin-Gsao (1911–1976 CE). Dr. Yang, Jwing-Ming's White Crane master.

chi (qi). The energy pervading the universe, including the energy circulating in the human body.

chi kung (qigong). The gongfu of qi, which means the study of qi.

chize (L-5). Cubit march. The name of an acupuncture cavity that belongs to the lung channel.

chong mai. Thrusting vessel. One of the eight extraordinary qi vessels.

chongyang (S-42). Pouring yang. The name of an acupuncture cavity that belongs to the stomach channel.

dadun (Li-1). Great honesty. The name of an acupuncture cavity that belongs to the liver channel.

dai mai. Girdle (or belt) vessel. One of the eight qi vessels.

daling (P-7). Big tomb. The name of an acupuncture cavity that belongs to the pericardium channel.

dan. Elixir. In qigong society, elixir usually implies the qi circulating in the body that maintains the health and increases longevity.

dan tian. Literally, "field of elixir." Locations in the body that are able to store and generate qi (elixir) in the body. The upper, middle, and lower dan tian are located, respectively, between the eyebrows, at the solar plexus, and a few inches below the navel.

dan tian qi. Usually, the qi that is converted from original essence and stored in the lower dan tian. This qi is considered "water qi" and is able to calm the body. Also called xian tian qi (preheaven qi).

Dao. The "way," by implication the "natural way."

Dao De Jing. *Morality Classic* or *Classic on the Virtue of the Dao,* written by Lao Zi (604–531 BCE).

dian. To point or to press.

dian mai (dim mak). Mai means "the blood vessel" (xue mai) or "the qi channel" (qi mai). Dian mai means "to press the blood vessel or qi channel."

dian qi. Dian means "electricity" and so dian qi means "electrical energy" (electricity). In China, a word is often placed before "qi" to identify the different kinds of energy.

dian xue. Dian means "to point and exert pressure" and xue means "the cavities." Dian xue refers to those qin na techniques that specialize in attacking acupuncture cavities to immobilize or kill an opponent.

dian xue an mo. A Chinese massage technique in which the acupuncture cavities are stimulated through pressure. Dian xue massage is also called acupressure and is the root of Japanese shiatsu.

dim mak (dian mai). Cantonese for dian mai.

du mai. Usually translated "governing vessel." One of the eight extraordinary vessels.

dubi (S-35 or M-LE-16). This cavity is called "eyes of knee" (xiyan). It is on the stomach channel and is also called "calf's nose" (dubi) when classified as one of the miscellaneous points.

feng shi. Literally, "wind moisture," often translated as "rheumatism" in Western society.

fengchi (GB-20). Pool of wind. The name of an acupuncture cavity that belongs to the gall bladder channel.

fengfu (Gv-16). Wind's dwelling. The name of an acupuncture cavity that belongs to the governing vessel.

Gao, Tao. Master Yang, Jwing-Ming's first taijiquan master.

gong (kung). Energy or hard work.

gongfu (kung fu). Means "energy-time." Anything that will take time and energy to learn or to accomplish is called gongfu.

guan jie yan. Literally, "joint inflammation" and means arthritis.

Han dynasty. A dynasty in Chinese history (206 BCE–221 CE).

Han, Ching-Tang. A well-known Chinese martial artist. Master Han is also Dr. Yang, Jwing-Ming's Long Fist grandmaster.

heding (M-LE-27). Crane's top. The name of an acupuncture cavity that belongs to the miscellaneous points.

hegu (LI-4). Adjoining valleys. The name of an acupuncture cavity that belongs to the large intestine channel.

huantiao (GB-30). Encircling leap. An acupuncture point that belongs to the gall bladder primary qi channel.

jianjing (GB-21). Shoulder well. The name of an acupuncture cavity that belongs to the gall bladder primary qi channel.

jianliao (TB-14). Shoulder seam. The name of an acupuncture cavity that belongs to the triple burner channel.

jianqian (M-UE-48). Shoulder front. The name of an acupuncture cavity that belongs to the miscellaneous points. This cavity is also called jianneiling (shoulder's inner tomb).

jiexi (S-41). Release stream. The name of an acupuncture cavity that belongs to the stomach primary qi channel.

jin. Means "tendons."

Jin, Shao-Feng. Dr. Yang, Jwing-Ming's White Crane grandmaster.

jing. Essence. The most refined part of anything.

jing. Calm and silent.

jing. Channels. Sometimes translated "meridian." Refers to the twelve organ-related "rivers" that circulate qi throughout the body.

jubi (N-UE-10). Raise arm. The name of an acupuncture cavity that belongs to the "new points."

jugu (LI-16). Great bone. The name of an acupuncture cavity that belongs to the large intestine channel.

juliao (GB-29). Stationary seam. The name of an acupuncture cavity that belongs to the gall bladder primary qi channel.

kan. One of the eight trigrams.

kung (gong). Means energy or hard work.

kung fu (gongfu). Literally, energy-time. Any study, learning, or practice that requires much patience, energy, and time to complete. Because practicing Chinese martial arts requires a great deal of time and energy, Chinese martial arts are commonly called gongfu.

kunlun (B-60). Kunlun mountains. The name of an acupuncture cavity that belongs to the bladder channel.

Lao Zi. The creator of Daoism, also called Li Er.

laogong (P-8). Labor's palace. The name of an acupuncture cavity that belongs to the pericardium channel. The laogong is located in the center of the palm.

Li, Mao-Ching. Dr. Yang, Jwing-Ming's Long Fist master.

linqi (GB-41). Near tears. The name of an acupuncture cavity that belongs to the gall bladder channel.

luo. The small qi channels that branch out from the primary qi channels and are connected to the skin and to the bone marrow.

mai. Means "vessel" or "qi channel."

mingmen (Gv-4). Life's door. The name of an acupuncture cavity that belongs to the governing vessel.

nei dan. Literally, internal elixir. A form of qigong in which qi (the elixir) is built up in the body and spread out to the limbs.

qi (chi). The general definition of qi is: universal energy, including heat, light, and electromagnetic energy. A narrower definition of qi refers to the energy circulating in human or animal bodies. A current popular model is that the qi circulating in the human body is bioelectric in nature.

qigong (chi kung). Gong means gongfu (literally, "energy-time"). Therefore, qigong means study, research, and practices related to qi.

qihai (Co-6). Sea of qi. The name of an acupuncture cavity that belongs to the conception vessel.

qihaishu (B-24). Sea of qi hollow. The name of an acupuncture cavity that belongs to the bladder channel.

quchi (LI-11). Crooked pool. The name of an acupuncture cavity that belongs to the large intestine channel.

quze (P-3). Crooked marsh. The name of an acupuncture cavity that belongs to the pericardium channel.

ren mai. Conception vessel. One of the eight extraordinary vessels.

sanjian (LI-3). Between three. The name of an acupuncture cavity that belongs to the large intestine channel.

sanjiaoshu (B-22). Triple burner's hollow. The name of an acupuncture cavity that belongs to the bladder channel.

shang dan tian. Upper dan tian. Located at the third eye, it is the residence of the shen (spirit).

shangbaxie (M-UE-50). Upper eight evils. The name of an acupuncture cavity that belongs to the miscellaneous points.

shangliao (B-31). One of four cavities on each side of the sacrum that belongs to the bladder primary qi channel.

shaohai (H-3). Lesser sea. The name of an acupuncture cavity that belongs to the heart channel.

Shaolin Temple. A monastery located in Henan Province, China. The Shaolin Temple is well known because of its martial arts training.

shaoshang (L-11). Lesser merchant. The name of an acupuncture cavity that belongs to the lung channel.

Shaoze (SI-1). Lesser marsh. The name of an acupuncture cavity that belongs to the small intestine channel.

shen. Spirit. According to Chinese qigong, the shen resides at the upper dan tian (shang dan tian—the third eye).

shenmai (B-62). Extending vessel. The name of an acupuncture cavity that belongs to the bladder channel.

shenmen (H-7). Spirit's door. The name of an acupuncture cavity that belongs to the heart channel.

shenshu (B-23). Kidney's hollow. The name of an acupuncture cavity that belongs to the bladder qi channel.

shi er jing. The twelve primary qi channels in Chinese medicine.

shiqizhuixia (M-BW-25). Below the seventeenth vertebra. The name of an acupuncture cavity that belongs to the miscellaneous points.

shousanli (LI-10). Arm's three measures. The name of an acupuncture cavity that belongs to the large intestine channel.

si qi. Dead qi. The qi remaining in a dead body. Sometimes called "ghost qi" (gui qi).

sifeng (M-UE-9). Four seams. The name of an acupuncture cavity that belongs to the miscellaneous points.

taichong (Li-3). Great pouring. The name of an acupuncture cavity that belongs to the liver channel.

taijian (N-UE-11). Lift shoulder. The name of an acupuncture cavity that belongs to the new points.

taijiquan (tai chi chuan). A Chinese internal martial style that is based on the theory of taiji (grand ultimate).

Taipei. The capital city of Taiwan.

Taiwan. An island to the southeast of mainland China. Also known as Formosa.

Taiwan University. A well-known university located in northern Taiwan.

taixi (K-3). Great creek. The name of an acupuncture cavity that belongs to the kidney channel.

taiyuan (L-9). Great abyss. The name of an acupuncture cavity that belongs to the lung channel.

Tamkang. Name of a university in Taiwan.

Tamkang College Guoshu Club. A Chinese martial arts club founded by Dr. Yang when he was studying in Tamkang College.

tian. Heaven or sky. In ancient China, people believed that heaven was the most powerful natural energy in this universe.

tian qi. Heaven qi. It is now commonly used to mean the weather, as weather is governed by heaven qi.

tian shi. Heavenly timing. The repeated natural cycles generated by the heavens such as seasons, months, days, and hours.

tianzhu (B-10). Heaven's pillar. The name of an acupuncture cavity that belongs to the bladder channel.

tongli (H-5). Reaching the measure. The name of an acupuncture cavity that belongs to the heart channel.

tui na. Means "to push and grab." A category of Chinese massages for healing and injury treatment.

wai. External.

wai dan. External elixir. External qigong exercises in which a practitioner will build up the qi in his or her limbs and then lead it into the center of the body for nourishment.

wai dan qigong (wai dan chi kung). External elixir qigong. In wai dan qigong, a practitioner will generate qi to the limbs and then allow the qi to flow inward to nourish the internal organs.

wei qi. Protective qi or guardian qi. The qi at the surface of the body that generates a shield to protect the body from negative external influences such as colds.

weishang (N-LE-25). Above the commission. The name of an acupuncture cavity that belongs to the "new points."

weiyang (B-53). Commission the yang. The name of an acupuncture cavity that belongs to the bladder channel.

weizhong (B-54). Commission the middle. The name of an acupuncture cavity that belongs to the bladder primary qi channel.

Wilson Chen. Dr. Yang, Jwing-Ming's friend.

Wuji. Means "no extremity."

wuji qigong. A style of taiji qigong practice.

xi sui gong. Gongfu for marrow and brain washing qigong practice.

xi sui jing. Literally, washing marrow/brain classic, usually translated marrow/brain washing classic. A qigong training that specializes in leading qi to the marrow to cleanse it or to the brain to nourish the spirit for enlightenment. It is believed that xi sui jing training is the key to longevity and achieving spiritual enlightenment.

xia dan tian. Lower dan tian. Located in the lower abdomen, it is believed to be the residence of water qi (original qi).

xian tian qi. Prebirth qi or pre-heaven qi. Also called dan tian qi. The qi that is converted from original essence and is stored in the lower tian. Considered to be "water qi," it is able to calm the body.

xiangu (S-43). Sinking valley. The name of an acupuncture cavity that belongs to the stomach channel.

xiaohai (SI-8). Small sea. The name of an acupuncture cavity that belongs to the small intestine channel.

Xinzhu Xian. Birthplace of Dr. Yang, Jwing-Ming in Taiwan.

xiyangquan (GB-33). Knee's yang hinge. The name of an acupuncture cavity that belongs to the gall bladder channel.

yamen (Gv-15). Door of muteness. The name of an acupuncture cavity that belongs to the governing vessel.

yang. In Chinese philosophy, the active, positive, masculine polarity. In Chinese medicine, yang means excessive, overactive, overheated. The yang organs are the gall bladder, small intestine, large intestine, stomach, bladder, and triple burner.

Yang, Jwing-Ming. Author of this book.

Yang, Xie-Jin. Name of Dr. Yang, Jwing-Ming's mother.

yangchi (TB-4). Pool of yang. The name of an acupuncture cavity that belongs to the triple burner channel.

yanglao (SI-6). Nourish the old. The name of an acupuncture cavity that belongs to the small intestine channel.

yangxi (LI-5). Yang creek. The name of an acupuncture cavity that belongs to the large intestine channel.

yaoqi (M-BW-29). Lower back's miscellany. The name of an acupuncture cavity that belongs to the miscellaneous points.

yaoshu (Gv-2). Lower back's hollow. The name of an acupuncture cavity that belongs to the governing vessel.

yaoyangquan (Gv-3). Lumber yang's hinge. The name of an acupuncture cavity that belongs to the governing vessel.

yi. Mind. Specifically, the mind that is generated by clear thinking and judgment and that is able to make you calm, peaceful, and wise.

Yi Jin Jing. Literally, changing muscle/tendon classic, usually called *The Muscle/Tendon Changing Classic.* Credited to Da Mo around 550 CE, this work discusses wai dan qigong training for strengthening the physical body.

yi shou dan tian. Keep your yi on your lower dan tian. In qigong training, you keep your mind at the lower dan tian in order to build up qi. When you are circulating your qi, you always lead your qi back to your lower dan tian before you stop.

yi yi yin qi. Use your yi (wisdom mind) to lead your qi. A qigong technique. Yi cannot be pushed, but it can be led. This is best done with the yi.

yin. In Chinese philosophy, the passive, negative, feminine polarity. In Chinese medicine, yin means deficient. The yin organs are the heart, lungs, liver, kidneys, spleen, and pericardium.

yinbai (Sp-l). Hidden white. The name of an acupuncture cavity that belongs to the spleen channel.

yongquan (K-1). Bubbling well. Name of an acupuncture cavity belonging to the kidney primary qi channel.

yuan qi. Original qi. The qi created from the original essence inherited from your parents.

zhaohai (K-6). Shining sea. The name of an acupuncture cavity that belongs to the kidney channel.

zhen dan tian. The real dan tian, which is located at the physical center of gravity.

zhibian (B-49). An acupuncture cavity belonging to the bladder primary qi channel.

zhiyin (B-67). End of yin. The name of an acupuncture cavity that belongs to the bladder channel.

zhong dan tian. Middle dan tian. Located in the area of the solar plexus, it is the residence of fire qi.

zhongliao (B-33). Middle seam. One of four cavities on each side of the sacrum that belongs to the bladder primary qi channel.

zhongzhu (TB-3). Middle island. The name of an acupuncture cavity that belongs to the triple burner channel.

About the Author

Yang, Jwing-Ming, PhD (楊俊敏博士)

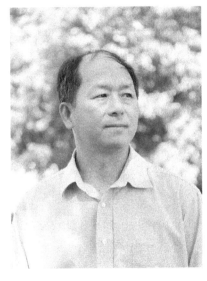

Dr. Yang, Jwing-Ming was born on August 11, 1946, in Xinzhu Xian, Taiwan, Republic of China. He started his wushu (gongfu or kung fu) training at the age of fifteen under Shaolin White Crane (Shaolin Bai He) Master Cheng, Gin-Gsao (曾金灶). Master Cheng originally learned taizuquan from his grandfather when he was a child. When Master Cheng was fifteen years old, he started learning White Crane from Master Jin, Shao-Feng (金紹峰) and followed him for twenty-three years until Master Jin's death.

In thirteen years of study (1961–1974) under Master Cheng, Dr. Yang became an expert in the White Crane style of Chinese martial arts, which includes both the use of bare hands and various weapons, such as saber, staff, spear, trident, two short rods, and many others. With the same master, he also studied White Crane qigong, qin na (chin na), tui na, and dian xue massages and herbal treatment.

At sixteen, Dr. Yang began the study of Yang-style taijiquan under Master Kao Tao (高濤). He later continued his study of taijiquan under Master Li, Mao-Ching (李茂清) and was also a student with Mr. Wilson Chen (陳威伸) in Taipei. Master Li learned his taijiquan from the well-known Master Han, Ching-Tang (韓慶堂), and Mr. Chen learned his taijiquan from Master Chang, Xiang-San (張詳三). From this further practice, Dr. Yang was able to master the taiji bare-hand sequence, pushing hands, the two-man fighting sequence, taiji sword, taiji saber, and taiji qigong.

When Dr. Yang was eighteen years old, he entered Tamkang College in Taipei Xian to study physics. In college, he began the study of traditional Shaolin Long Fist (changquan or chang chuan) with Master Li, Mao-Ching at the Tamkang College Guoshu Club, 1964–1968, and eventually became an assistant instructor under Master Li. In 1971 he completed his MS degree in physics at the National Taiwan University and then served in the Chinese Air Force from 1971 to 1972. In the service, Dr. Yang taught physics at the Junior Academy of the Chinese Air Force while also teaching wushu. After being honorably discharged in 1972, he returned to Tamkang College to teach physics and resumed study under Master Li, Mao-Ching. From Master Li, Dr. Yang learned Northern-style wushu, which includes bare-hand and kicking techniques as well as numerous weapons.

In 1974 Dr. Yang came to the United States to study mechanical engineering at Purdue University. At the request of a few students, Dr. Yang began to teach gongfu (kung fu), which resulted in the establishment of the Purdue University Chinese Kung Fu Research Club in the spring of 1975. While at Purdue, Dr. Yang also taught college-credit courses in taijiquan. In May 1978, he was awarded a PhD in mechanical engineering by Purdue.

In 1980 Dr. Yang moved to Houston to work for Texas Instruments. While in Houston, he founded Yang's Shaolin Kung Fu Academy, which was eventually taken over by his disciple, Mr. Jeffery Bolt, after Dr. Yang moved to Boston in 1982. Dr. Yang founded Yang's Martial Arts Academy in Boston on October 1, 1982.

In January 1984, he gave up his engineering career to devote more time to research, writing, and teaching. In March 1986, he purchased property in the Jamaica Plain area of Boston to be used as the headquarters of the new organization, Yang's Martial Arts Association (YMAA). The organization expanded to become a division of Yang's Oriental Arts Association, Inc. (YOAA).

In 2008 Dr. Yang began the nonprofit YMAA California Retreat Center. This training facility in rural California is where selected students enroll in a five-year residency to learn Chinese martial arts.

Dr. Yang has been involved in traditional Chinese wushu since 1961, studying Shaolin White Crane (bai he), Shaolin Long Fist (changquan), and taijiquan under several different masters. He has taught for almost fifty years: seven years in Taiwan, five years at Purdue University, two years in Houston, twenty-six years in Boston, and more than eight years at the YMAA California Retreat Center. He has taught seminars all over the world, sharing his knowledge of Chinese martial arts and qigong in Argentina, Austria, Barbados, Botswana, Belgium, Bermuda, Brazil, Canada, China, Chile, England, Egypt, France, Germany, Hungary, Iceland, Iran, Ireland, Italy, Latvia, Mexico, the Netherlands, New Zealand, Poland, Portugal, Saudi Arabia, South Africa, Spain, Switzerland, and Venezuela.

Since 1986 YMAA has become an international organization, which currently includes more than fifty schools located in Argentina, Belgium, Canada, Chile, France, Hungary, Iran, Ireland, Italy, New Zealand, Poland, Portugal, South Africa, Sweden, the United Kingdom, the United States, and Venezuela.

Many of Dr. Yang's books and videos have been translated into other languages, such as French, Italian, Spanish, Polish, Czech, Bulgarian, Russian, German, and Hungarian.

Books and Videos by Dr. Yang, Jwing-Ming

Books Alphabetical

Analysis of Shaolin Chin Na, 2nd ed. YMAA Publication Center, 1987, 2004

Ancient Chinese Weapons: A Martial Artist's Guide, 2nd ed. YMAA Publication Center, 1985, 1999

Arthritis Relief: Chinese Qigong for Healing & Prevention, 2nd ed. YMAA Publication Center, 1991, 2005

Back Pain Relief: Chinese Qigong for Healing and Prevention, 2nd ed. YMAA Publication Center, 1997, 2004

Baguazhang: Theory and Applications, 2nd ed. YMAA Publication Center, 1994, 2008

Comprehensive Applications of Shaolin Chin Na: The Practical Defense of Chinese Seizing Arts. YMAA Publication Center, 1995

Essence of Shaolin White Crane. YMAA Publication Center, 1996

How to Defend Yourself. YMAA Publication Center, 1992

Introduction to Ancient Chinese Weapons. Unique Publications, Inc., 1985

Meridian Qigong, YMAA Publication Center, 2016

Northern Shaolin Sword, 2nd ed. YMAA Publication Center, 1985, 2000

Pain-Free Joints: 46 Simple Qigong Movements for Arthritis Healing and Prevention. YMAA Publication Center, 2017

Qigong for Health and Martial Arts, 2nd ed. YMAA Publication Center, 1995, 1998

Qigong Massage: Fundamental Techniques for Health and Relaxation, 2nd ed. YMAA Publication Center, 1992, 2005

Qigong Meditation: Embryonic Breathing. YMAA Publication Center, 2003

Qigong Meditation: Small Circulation. YMAA Publication Center, 2006

Qigong, the Secret of Youth: Da Mo's Muscle/Tendon Changing and Marrow/Brain Washing Qigong, 2nd ed. YMAA Publication Center, 1989, 2000

Root of Chinese Qigong: Secrets of Qigong Training, 2nd ed. YMAA Publication Center, 1989, 2004

Shaolin Chin Na. Unique Publications, Inc., 1980

Shaolin Long Fist Kung Fu. Unique Publications, Inc., 1981

Simple Qigong Exercises for Health: The Eight Pieces of Brocade, 3rd ed. YMAA Publication Center, 1988, 1997, 2013

Tai Chi Ball Qigong: For Health and Martial Arts. YMAA Publication Center, 2010

Tai Chi Chin Na: The Seizing Art of Taijiquan, 2nd ed. YMAA Publication Center, 1995, 2014

Tai Chi Chuan Classical Yang Style: The Complete Long Form and Qigong, 2nd ed. YMAA Publication Center, 1999, 2010

Tai Chi Chuan Martial Applications, 2nd ed. YMAA Publication Center, 1986, 1996

Tai Chi Chuan Martial Power, 3rd ed. YMAA Publication Center, 1986, 1996, 2015

Tai Chi Chuan: Classical Yang Style, 2nd ed. YMAA Publication Center, 1999, 2010

Tai Chi Qigong: The Internal Foundation of Tai Chi Chuan, 2nd ed. rev. YMAA Publication Center, 1997, 1990, 2013

Tai Chi Secrets of the Ancient Masters: Selected Readings with Commentary. YMAA Publication Center, 1999

Tai Chi Secrets of the Wû and Li Styles: Chinese Classics, Translation, Commentary. YMAA Publication Center, 2001

Tai Chi Secrets of the Wu Style: Chinese Classics, Translation, Commentary. YMAA Publication Center, 2002

Tai Chi Secrets of the Yang Style: Chinese Classics, Translation, Commentary. YMAA Publication Center, 2001

Tai Chi Sword Classical Yang Style: The Complete Long Form, Qigong, and Applications, 2nd ed. YMAA Publication Center, 1999, 2014

Taijiquan Theory of Dr. Yang, Jwing-Ming: The Root of Taijiquan. YMAA Publication Center, 2003

The Pain-Free Back: 54 Qigong Movements for Healing and Prevention. YMAA Publication Center, 2017

Xingyiquan: Theory and Applications, 2nd ed. YMAA Publication Center, 1990, 2003

Yang Style Tai Chi Chuan. Unique Publications, Inc., 1981

Videos Alphabetical

Advanced Practical Chin Na in Depth. YMAA Publication Center, 2010

Analysis of Shaolin Chin Na. YMAA Publication Center, 2004

Baguazhang (Eight Trigrams Palm Kung Fu). YMAA Publication Center, 2005

Chin Na in Depth: Courses 1–4. YMAA Publication Center, 2003

Chin Na in Depth: Courses 5–8. YMAA Publication Center, 2003

Chin Na in Depth: Courses 9–12. YMAA Publication Center, 2003

Five Animal Sports Qigong. YMAA Publication Center, 2008

Knife Defense: Traditional Techniques. YMAA Publication Center, 2011

Meridian Qigong. YMAA Publication Center, 2015

Neigong. YMAA Publication Center, 2015

Northern Shaolin Sword. YMAA Publication Center, 2009

Qigong Massage. YMAA Publication Center, 2005

Saber Fundamental Training. YMAA Publication Center, 2008

Shaolin Kung Fu Fundamental Training. YMAA Publication Center, 2004

Shaolin Long Fist Kung Fu: Basic Sequences. YMAA Publication Center, 2005

Shaolin Saber Basic Sequences. YMAA Publication Center, 2007

Shaolin Staff Basic Sequences. YMAA Publication Center, 2007

Shaolin White Crane Gong Fu Basic Training: Courses 1 & 2. YMAA Publication Center, 2003

Shaolin White Crane Gong Fu Basic Training: Courses 3 & 4. YMAA Publication Center, 2008

Shaolin White Crane Hard and Soft Qigong. YMAA Publication Center, 2003

Shuai Jiao: Kung Fu Wrestling. YMAA Publication Center, 2010

Simple Qigong Exercises for Arthritis Relief. YMAA Publication Center, 2007

Simple Qigong Exercises for Back Pain Relief. YMAA Publication Center, 2007

Simple Qigong Exercises for Health: The Eight Pieces of Brocade. YMAA Publication Center, 2003

Staff Fundamental Training: Solo Drills and Matching Practice. YMAA Publication Center, 2007

Sword Fundamental Training. YMAA Publication Center, 2009

Tai Chi Ball Qigong: Courses 1 & 2. YMAA Publication Center, 2006

Tai Chi Ball Qigong: Courses 3 & 4. YMAA Publication Center, 2007

Tai Chi Chuan: Classical Yang Style. YMAA Publication Center, 2003

Tai Chi Fighting Set: 2-Person Matching Set. YMAA Publication Center, 2006

Tai Chi Pushing Hands: Courses 1 & 2. YMAA Publication Center, 2005

Tai Chi Pushing Hands: Courses 3 & 4. YMAA Publication Center, 2006

Tai Chi Qigong. YMAA Publication Center, 2005

Tai Chi Sword, Classical Yang Style. YMAA Publication Center, 2005

Tai Chi Symbol: Yin/Yang Sticking Hands. YMAA Publication Center, 2008

Taiji 37 Postures Martial Applications. YMAA Publication Center, 2008

Taiji Chin Na in Depth. YMAA Publication Center, 2009

Taiji Saber: Classical Yang Style. YMAA Publication Center, 2008

Taiji Wrestling: Advanced Takedown Techniques. YMAA Publication Center, 2008

Understanding Qigong, DVD 1: What Is Qigong? The Human Qi Circulatory System. YMAA Publication Center, 2006

Understanding Qigong, DVD 2: Key Points of Qigong & Qigong Breathing. YMAA Publication Center, 2006

Understanding Qigong, DVD 3: Embryonic Breathing. YMAA Publication Center, 2007

Understanding Qigong, DVD 4: Four Seasons Qigong. YMAA Publication Center, 2007

Understanding Qigong, DVD 5: Small Circulation. YMAA Publication Center, 2007

Understanding Qigong, DVD 6: Martial Arts Qigong Breathing. YMAA Publication Center, 2007

Xingyiquan: Twelve Animals Kung Fu and Applications. YMAA Publication Center, 2008

Yang Tai Chi for Beginners. YMAA Publication Center, 2012

YMAA 25-Year Anniversary. YMAA Publication Center, 2009

Index

weakness of the internal organs, 5

Western medicine, xv, xvii, xviii, 1, 4–5, 8, 16–17, 24, 26–27

wisdom mind, 32, 34, 36, 118

wrists, xviii, xix, 69, 72, 84–85, 87–89, 98

wuji qigong, 116

xi sui jing, 51, 116

xingyiquan, 124, 126

Yellow Emperor (Huang Di)

yi, 36, 41, 51, 55, 76, 117–118

yi jin jing, 51, 117

yin and yang, 20

yongquan, 47–48, 74, 118

BOOKS FROM YMAA

DVDS FROM YMAA

more products available from . . .
YMAA Publication Center, Inc. 楊氏東方文化出版中心

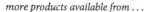

1-800-669-8892 • info@ymaa.com • www.ymaa.com